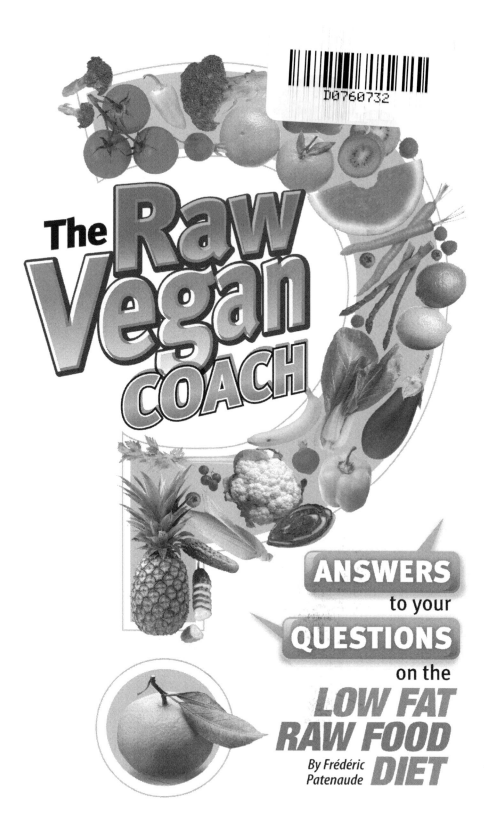

The Raw Vegan COACH

ANSWERS to your **QUESTIONS** on the **LOW FAT RAW FOOD DIET**

By Frédéric Patenaude

D0760732

Important Medical Disclaimer

The information in this book does not constitute medical or health advice, but it simply intends to share the personal experiences of Frederic Patenaude with healthful living.

Frederic Patenaude does not provide any medical opinions or health advice. If you have questions regarding specific medical or healthcare matters, you should speak directly with your doctor, pharmacist, or licensed healthcare provider. The information contained in this book is not intended to replace the advice of a licensed healthcare provider.

Copyright Information

Published by:

FredericPatenaude.Com
8605 Santa Monica Blvd #6370
Los Angeles, California 90069
USA

www.fredericpatenaude.com

www.rawvegan.com

www.rawstarterkit.com

www.dowhatyoulove.com

To contact us, please go to www.replytofred.com

Table of Contents

Chapter 1:
Defining the High-Fruit, Low-Fat Diet

One of the most common questions that I receive on the raw food diet is "What do you eat?"

When I tell people that a raw food diet is basically a diet of fruits and vegetables, the simplicity of my answer confuses them.

"But, Fred, it's not possible to eat just fruits and vegetables! Where do you get your protein? You must be always hungry!"

I go on to explain that as long as you consume enough fruits and vegetables, in terms of total calories, you will get enough vitamins, minerals, and, yes, even protein!

But, when I tell people how much fruit they should be eating to get those calories, they are often shocked by the quantities.

Most cultures view fruit as a mere snack or an afterthought to the meal, but not an actual item of sustenance. Therefore, the quantities consumed are ridiculously small: half a grapefruit, one orange, a few slices of watermelon, etc.

Most cooked foods are also extremely concentrated. They pack a lot of calories in a small package! For example, a meal of one burger with fries and a drink can easily represent 800 to 1000 calories, which is about half of what the average person really needs in a day. To get the same calories from fruit, you would need to eat 8 to 10 bananas or 5 to 6 large mangoes.

A big trap of the raw food diet is in not understanding the quantities of fruits and vegetables that are necessary to consume to thrive and the proper amounts of concentrated fatty foods, such as nuts, seeds, avocados, and oils, which must be added. However, these fatty foods should only be consumed in small quantities and not at every meal. Most raw-foodists don't realize that since vegetables don't contain many calories, and fruit must be consumed in large quantities to provide significant energy, that most of their calories actually come from fat.

It's not rare for a raw-foodist to have a fat intake that is about 60% or more of fat by total calories, which is at least twice the upper limit of even relatively conservative, official nutritional recommendations.

So this chapter is dedicated to the raw food controversy around fruit and the low-fat, raw vegan diet.

25 Bananas a Day

Q: *Some people eat 25 bananas a day on this diet. It seems a bit extreme. Do I have to do that?*

A: The idea of eating 25 bananas in a day seems to strike some people as particularly unhealthy. So let's settle the controversy:
You DON'T have to eat 25 bananas in a day.

If you're going to eat all raw food, you just have to eat enough calories to meet your needs. If you need 2000 calories a day, like most sedentary to moderately active people, then 25 bananas is going to be too much.

If you need 5000 calories, because you're a training athlete, then 25 bananas are going to cover only 50% of your needs. You don't have to eat just bananas. This is one example to give you a visual idea. You can eat a combination of fruits, vegetables, nuts, seeds, etc. and spread them out over several meals.

Eating Too Many Fruits and Vegetables

Q: *I was feeling really comfortable with the idea of eating a mostly fruit diet, as long as greens, nuts and seeds were included, too, but then I read an article that's really thrown me. The author states, "Any food in large quantities is going to harm you." For example, if you go crazy on apples, carrots, or any other fruit or veggies, then it is going to throw your system out of balance and cause harm in the long run.*

A: What is a "large" quantity of fruits and vegetables? It might look large compared to what most people are used to eating, but it's actually a "normal" quantity. I, personally, don't see how eating lots of fruits and vegetables can be bad for you if the diet is otherwise balanced and provides every nutrient that you need. There are sometimes problems associated with eating too much of one particular food, such as acidic fruits, for example. In general, it's very difficult to overeat on one type of fresh, raw fruit or vegetable. Personally, I'm going to stick with the idea of fruits and vegetables in "adequate" quantities being the healthiest foods.

Many people have eaten large quantities of the same fruit for days or even weeks with no ill effects. Your body has lots of stores that will not get thrown out of whack if you eat a large quantity of one fruit or vegetable for a short period of time.

I think they are misleading you to think that a day or a week on the same food could cause harm in the long run. Many rural people in Europe and Asia eat large amounts of the same fruits, vegetables, rice, and beans week in and week out, and they are some of the healthiest people in the world.

The body is highly intelligent and won't let you throw it out of whack just by eating large quantities of fruits and vegetables. It's what your body was designed for.

What the author should have said is that concentrated or toxic foods in large quantities are bad for you. For example, food like meat, bread, dairy, sprouts, bitter greens, refined oils, dried fruits and nuts, in large quantities may cause harm.

Fruits and vegetables are water rich and not concentrated, so you will have no problem digesting them.

There are a few exceptions to watch out for, such as:

- *Very acidic fruits (such as acid pineapple, acid kiwis, etc)*

- *Dates and very sugary fruits*

- *Astringent fruits (such as unripe persimmon)*

Eating When Hungry

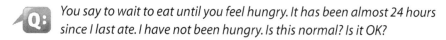

Q: *You say to wait to eat until you feel hungry. It has been almost 24 hours since I last ate. I have not been hungry. Is this normal? Is it OK?*

A: In my book, The Raw Secrets, I described in detail the difference between true, genuine hunger and false "appetite" or hunger. This was more to enable the reader to recognize these differences and more accurately judge if the diet they are on is really working.

That being said, I don't recommend waiting to eat every time until you are absolutely, genuinely hungry.

I recommend that you avoid all the foods and substances that trigger false hunger (such as salt, condiments, spices, sauces, etc.) and exercise daily to create a true demand for food. But, once that's done, eat at regular times, even if you are not ravenously hungry all the time. I find that, for myself, the most important thing to do to experience true hunger more frequently is to exercise regularly.

If you are going 24 hours between eating, and you are not trying to fast, your body could be thinking that you are fasting and not ask for food.

Don't eat when you feel sick or tired, but do give your body enough fuel when you need to work and be active.

Four Pounds of Fruit a Day

Q: *You suggest eating four pounds of fruits a day. How do I weigh the oranges and grapefruits? Should I weigh them with the skin or without? Some big oranges and grapefruits are heavy because of their very thick skin. How would I do it?*

A: The suggestion of 4 pounds a day is a strict minimum to get started on the raw food diet, but that is nowhere near the amounts necessary for optimal health for most people.

Instead of weighing your food, it's far better to measure food consumption by calories, because some fruits have much more calories per serving than others. The idea is to get most of your calories from fruit.

If you need to, log your calories at fitday.com or nutridiary.com to make sure you are getting enough calories from fruits and vegetables before you can visually assess how much you would need to eat every day.

Fruit Addiction Problem?

Q: *I have been eating mostly raw for the past several months. I fell off the wagon and started eating cooked foods. I was overeating terribly to the point of extreme discomfort. I have finally returned to all raw. However, I feel I have a fruit addiction problem. I get tired if I do not consume some fruit after 3 to 4 hours. I often find myself eating when I am not hungry or after 7 p.m. (which I never used to do). Can you make any suggestions? I know I am eating far too much fruit and subsequently too much sugar. I am angry with myself, and I have great trouble controlling my desires to eat more fruit. Any help would be greatly appreciated.*

A: I find it strange that you use the term "fruit addiction". If your body demands something, does that mean that you are "addicted"? Your body needs carbohydrates to run and fruits are the best source of whole, unrefined carbohydrates. Are all humans "addicted" to food because they need to eat it?

I seriously doubt that you are eating too much fruit. In fact, all of those symptoms are actually most likely caused by not eating enough fruit. You're feeling tired from low blood sugar, and you are eating later because you have not consumed enough calories to sustain your needs during the day.

Essentially, I recommend eating enough fruit at one meal so that you are satisfied for several hours afterwards. Eating every 3-5 hours is normal when eating low calorie, water rich foods. If you were eating every 1-2 hours, you would not be consuming enough calories, by far, at each meal. Since I do not know the details of your diet, it would be hard for me to make any other suggestions.

Fruit Ripeness

Q: *How can you tell when a fruit is at the "ripe" point to be considered the most nutritionally nutritious (i.e., mangoes, melons, bananas, etc.)? Why are mangoes so hard to cut, and what is the woody part of the fruit? I have yet to buy a mango that doesn't get wasted, because I cannot cut through the woody part. They are pretty expensive for so much waste.*

A: Every fruit is different, but most fruits are ripe when they are soft and smell sweet. That is also their nutritional peak. Bananas are ripe when they start to get some brown spots (although that can be different for some exotic varieties.) Melons are ripe when they are slightly soft at the ends and smell sweet. Mangoes should be soft and juicy, and certainly not hard like you have described. If they are hard, they are not yet ripe. Of course, don't eat the center pit. Cut around it on both sides. There are some varieties of mangoes that have smaller pits than others as well. There are many videos on YouTube showing how to cut a mango. Most people cut off the main fleshy sides and scoop the flesh from the peel.

Fruitarian is Fruit Only?

Q: *Is a fruitarian diet a diet of fruit only?*

A: There seems to be some confusion as to what a "high-fruit diet" is. First, what is a fruit? Nutritionally speaking, we are talking about sweet fruits, such as bananas, oranges, peaches, melons, mangoes, etc.

Even though avocados, tomatoes, and squash are also fruit, botanically speaking, we don't classify them as such, because, nutritionally speaking, they are vegetables.

Fatty foods and nuts form their own category.

Greens also can be seen as a separate category.

All of the fresh fruits and vegetables can and should be included in the raw diet. An abundance of greens and vegetables should be consumed as well.

But because vegetables are low in calories, if you eat 100% raw, then it's necessary that the bulk of your calories will come from fruit.

But that doesn't mean you're only eating fruit.

Some people choose to eat 100% fruit only. However, the term fruitarian generally means that the person eats mostly fruit, including some greens, nuts, or vegetables as well.

How to Make Green Smoothies

Q: *I'm very eager to start drinking green smoothies, but I have a question about how to make one. The percentage of fruit to greens is recommended to be 60/40. I was wondering if this is by percent weight or percent volume.*

For example, if I weighed out 60 grams of fruit and 40 grams of greens, would this be correct? Or do I fill the blender 60% with fruit and the other 40% with greens (which would be the percent of volume)?

If it weren't for your e-zines, I know I wouldn't be receiving enough education about the raw foods diet! Thank you so much for everything.

A: It's approximate, based on what you put in the blender. I don't rely on those ratios. I use more fruit myself. Usually, for 4 bananas, I'll put about 2 cups of greens. Each green has a different taste. Thus, you might only put 1 or 2 leaves of kale or dandelion greens, but you might add more spinach or romaine because of their milder taste.

Experiment! Try out some recipes. Change up the ratios and find one that you really enjoy.

If you really enjoy it, you'll drink more of it!

High-Fat or High-Fruit

 Hi, Fred! I think that your article on which raw diet to follow, high-fat or high-fruit, is misleading. It is entirely possible to thrive on a low-fat, plant-based, raw diet with minimal fruit, such as the Hippocrates diet that is recommended by Dr Gabriel Cousens.

I agree that the high-fat, raw diet can be problematic, but there are other ways to go low fat, raw food without eating vast amounts of fruit. You neglect to mention these, and I think that for people who do not have the benefit of a long standing, evidence based relationship with raw food, such as myself, it is too simplistic to divide these diets into only two options. Confusion could indeed reign.

In the Hippocrates regime, for example, approximately 10 to 15% of calories come from fat, and the diet limits fruit to 4-6 servings per WEEK, which is plenty for most people. I would also contend that it is sufficient for athletes as well, for I have coached several athletes who have done quite well with this regime.

I do not believe that there is "only one way and that's my way", but I do think that you should inform your readers that there are other ways to go with the raw diet than either high-fat or high-fruit. This amounts to scaremongering, which, ultimately, serves no-one.

I respect your opinion, but I would like to point out a big mistake that you're making in your statement.

You say that it's possible to thrive on a "low-fat", raw diet that contains "minimal fruit".

I would like to see how that works out in practice, because, from my nutritional training, this is simply not possible.

If you want a raw food diet, you will need to get most of your calories from two sources:

- *Fruit*

- *Fatty foods (avocados, nuts, oils, etc.)*

Vegetables have a low-caloric density. If you do not believe me, just check how many heads of lettuce or carrots you would need to eat to get the 4000 calories that your athletes need.

The other possible sources in a raw diet for calories are things that no one really wants to eat:

- *Sprouted grains and beans (They are very dry and cannot be eaten on their own. They often need condiments and to be prepared.)*

- *Carrot juice and other high sugar vegetable juices*

It's also known that raw, sprouted grains and beans contain natural toxins that do not go away simply through the sprouting process. You can get seriously ill from eating them and, in fact, many people have.

As far as using carrot juice or similar carbohydrate foods, it defeats the purpose in the first place. Aren't you avoiding fruit, because you think too much sugar is bad for you?

When people go to some raw food, detox places, what they follow is a very low-calorie diet. This type of diet is one that's good for a short period to lose a lot of weight, which is what most people want when they go to these places. This place is not for athletes, nor is this diet sustainable for the long term for a 100% raw-foodist.

They'll be served watermelon juice, green juice, and sprouts. I do not know anyone that is able to maintain that regimen when they go back to their regular lives.

If you follow a low fat, raw food diet and you limit your fruit consumption to 4 to 6 servings per week, you are following a very low-calorie diet that is not sustainable.

Or you are possibly eating massive quantities of sprouted grains and beans, which most people:

- *Wouldn't possibly *want* to do, and/or*

- *Would eventually get sick from because of the natural enzyme-inhibitors found in those foods.*

So these people are either under-eating on calories, which will only be sustainable in the short term, or they are going to be eating cooked carbohydrates or fats, which are not healthier than natural fruit sugars.

So, if you really want to prove me wrong, why don't you come up with a weekly menu, and we'll analyze it?

We know that athletes require more calories, usually 4000 a day or more. And you said that your diet can work for athletes.

So, send me a 7-day menu that contains 4000 calories per day (enough for an athlete — because if an athlete cannot follow your diet… is it really healthy?) and:

- *Contains a maximum of 12% fat by calories*
  (which is the average of the figures you gave me),

- *Contains a maximum of 4 to 6 servings of fruit per week,*

- *Is completely raw, and*

- *Is something that a human being would actually want to follow?*
  In other words, don't include gallons of carrot juice or buckets of sprouted beans just to make up for the lack of calories.

In fact, this is an open challenge to anyone.

Also, please note that Hippocrates does not even advocate a 100% raw diet. They believe eating cooked foods, including grains, are better for health than fruit and often promote 80% raw as a lifestyle with a focus on sprouts, not even greens or vegetables.

Low-Fat Means "No-Fat"

Q: *What is the difference between a low-fat diet and a no-fat diet?*

A: Some people seem to think that a "low-fat" diet means a "no-fat" diet. I have received a lot of comments from people who told me that I was not clearly defining the difference between good fats and bad fats.

The point I am making is that an extremely high-fat diet is unhealthy, regardless of where the fat comes from. The average raw-foodist eats 60% of his calories from fat, which is 20% higher than the Standard American Diet.

Just reduce that percentage to 20%, and you'll already be on your way to good health. Does it have to be 10% or less? That's what Dr. Graham recommends after 25+ years of experience.

A study of the three-longest lived cultures in the world showed that they eat, on average, 15% of their calories from fat. My recommendations: reduce the fat progressively, and increase the fruits and vegetables. Less than 15% is ideal.

There is so much marketing about good fats and bad fats that people are still thinking they need to eat a certain type of fat for a specific health benefit. The reason there is because so many marketing techniques are trying to offset the amount of unhealthy animal fats being consumed by the public by promoting "healthier" alternatives.

However, you can still enjoy delicious avocados, nuts, seeds, and even a tablespoon of olive oil on your salad once in a while, and it won't hurt you if you're on a low-fat diet. It's the overall picture that matters.

Question about Fat

 I'm wondering more and more about the promotion of raw fats in raw food diets. I'd like to know your opinion. Here's the type of advice we get:

- Eat 3 whole, young coconuts a day to feel energetic.

- Eat 2 to 3 avocados every single day to build muscle.

- Have 2 pockets of durian every day to live longer.

- Eat 3 to 4 spoonfuls of pure coconut oil per day to protect your heart.

- Do not forget to eat your 2 tablespoons of flax oil in the morning.

- A cup of raw almonds everyday will make your skin smooth as a baby.

Fat is "IN". I read this kind of advice all over the place now. In printed magazines, in Internet forums, from various diet gurus, in books, it looks like a vegan version of a FATkins diet. Aren't there physiological problems when eating that much fat even if it is from a "good" source? What would the effect be? What kind of problems can one expect with a diet high in fat? What is too high and too low? I would like to read your perspective about this. I seem to recall somewhere that you yourself ate way too many fats for a while in California and had to suffer some consequences. Am I remembering this right? What happened? Did you get sick somehow? Thanks for looking into questions like this and sharing your answers with all of us.

Most vegetarian experts agree with each other, saying that the optimal fat intake is between 10% and 15% of calories. That's about one small avocado per day, without oils or anything else. Rural Chinese people eat less than 15%. Primates eat less than 10%. The effects of eating too much fat are numerous: the blood becomes fattier, utilization of carbohydrates is impaired, and blood sugar is unstable. As sugar gets trapped in the blood stream, candida and fungus will proliferate. Less oxygen is available to the cells and sick cells cannot be destroyed as efficiently. More energy is spent on digesting large amounts of fat, and this can leave you tired and fatigued in the middle of the day. When eating a fruit-based diet with lots of vegetables and with some nuts and seeds (1-2 ounces a day or less), you cannot eat "too little" fat. 10-15% is plenty for your needs. Too high is anything above that, especially when you start to get above 20%. Most raw diets are about 50-70% fat. If you eliminate fruit from a raw diet, or limit it to 15%, your diet will be above 50-60% fat. You cannot get enough calories from vegetables to sustain yourself, so, inevitably, you will be eating nuts, avocados, oils, flax crackers, etc. When I lived in California, I became seriously ill from eating too many nuts and too much fat every day. Back in the late 90's, myself, as well as other well-known raw-foodists, ate anything as long as it was raw. We ended up eating large quantities of avocados and prepared nut dishes. I would get blood sugar swings from eating fruit. I was spaced out. I couldn't concentrate. I was tired most of the time. I started having severe dental problems (like cavities, gum issues, etc). Now that my diet is low in fat, I can eat a whole large honeydew melon and not get spaced out at all. I can eat 6 large mangoes and be perfectly okay. No problems with concentration either. Large quantities of fat do not work when eating moderate to large quantities of fruit. Keep your fat intake low, and you will have little to no issues with blood sugar, digestion, and concentration.

What is a High-Fat Meal?

Q: *Could you please give me an example of a raw meal that contains too much fat? I don't eat more than 1.5 avocados every two weeks or drink any nut milks. What are some other common raw foods that secretly contain too much fat?*

A: Nuts, seeds, oils, avocados, and durian contain a lot of fat. Too much fat would be in the diet, in general, not just one meal. But let's look at a high-fat meal, for example:

A big salad with a 2-4 Tablespoons of olive oil, slices of avocado, olives, and a handful of nuts.

This has way too many kinds of fat. Stick to one kind of fat at a time, once a day, or less. Even a salad with olive oil and nuts or nuts and avocado would be too much fat.

Other examples would be flax crackers with nut pate, raw breads, pizza, sun burgers, falafels, nachos with guacamole and macadamia sour cream, any raw dessert that uses nuts as a base for crust or dough, raw ice creams with nut milks, etc.

Any combination of raw food that mimics cooked food is usually based around nuts, avocado, and oils with little vegetables. These meals are not natural and are designed for things like taste, texture, appearance, etc., not for health and not for a sustainable lifestyle. So be careful not to base your diet around these complicated raw meals, and eat them sparingly (if at all).

What's the Difference between "Low-Fat" And "No-Fat"?

Q: *Thanks for the always thought-provoking comments and advice. I really look forward to your newsletters every week! My question from the last newsletter is: What is low-fat as opposed to no-fat (which is what it sounds like you are really espousing)? Are you really saying not to eat any fat at all? If you ARE saying a little fat is okay, can you define how much on a daily basis and what any 'good' fats might be?*

A: No-fat would be impossible to do, because all fruits and vegetables contain a certain percentage of fat naturally, even if you don't taste it. Check it out at www.fitday.com. Every fruit or vegetable you enter on that website has some fat, some protein, and mostly carbohydrates.

But, when we talk about a low-fat diet, we mean that there is little ADDED fat in the form of concentrated fatty foods, such as avocados, nuts, seeds, oils, etc. A little fat is okay, in the form of avocados, nuts, and seeds, and other fatty foods, such as durian and coconuts, but not at the same time and not in one day for an overall healthy diet. How much fat is "low-fat" really depends on how much food you eat. It's based on the total percentage of calories eaten. But I'd say that it's probably much LESS than you imagine. Most people who say or think that they are on a low-fat diet actually eat over 40% of their calories from fat when it comes down to it. Some even eat as high as 60%. To give you an example, if you eat 2000 calories per day, which is average for a woman who's a little active, then that would be about 1/2 avocado, OR a very small handful of nuts. If you're more active and eat more, then you could increase those quantities based on the percentage of total calories needed. Remember, that the diet should be low in fat "on average". So that means that some days you could eat a little more fat, and, some days, you could eat no fat at all. By no fat, I mean no concentrated fatty foods.

For example, today, I won't be eating any concentrated fatty foods. I'll only be eating fruits and vegetables. Tomorrow, I might have a little sliced avocado in a salad (with no other fat). Another day, I might have some fresh coconut or durian. It's much easier to eat a low-fat diet if you eat simply and avoid those combo raw recipes.

One Size Fits All

Q: *Some people have been accusing you of a "one-size fits all" philosophy. That you're right, while everybody else is wrong. They're saying that "there's no single answer that can benefit everybody. Something that cures person A can kill person B".*

A: I strongly disagree with that statement, and the way it's often being used. One thing that I really hate is people who can't take a stand on certain issues, either because they haven't done the research or can't come up with a conclusion.

The most "useful" piece of advice you'll often get is to "just do what works for you", which is open to a LOT of interpretation. I believe that there are basic principles that work for everybody, but there are some exceptions. Some things are true, and some things are not. And, yes, some things are somewhat in-between.

For example, as a general rule, we can say that fruit and vegetables are the healthiest, most appropriate foods that human beings can eat.

Are there exceptions? Of course. Some people are allergic to strawberries. Some people have no teeth and can't chew vegetables. In those cases, compromises can be made. The diet can be adapted. It's not this fixed, rigid thing that everybody must follow, or else!

I am very open-minded. In fact, I'm far from what you could call a "militant raw-foodist" by any definition. Just meet me in person, and you will see.

However, I will also take a stance on certain issues. I hate wishy-washy writings and advice, such as "just do what works for you", which ultimately doesn't help you in any way. You're still left lost and confused, looking for a real answer.

I believe certain things are TRUE, and I will let you know which ones and why. That doesn't mean that you have to agree with me. It's about more than food.

Some people have said: "It's about more than food. There's also the importance of exercise, peace of mind, etc. Some raw-foodists eat a perfect diet, and they still are not healthy."

I couldn't agree more. Yes, it's about more than food. But food is also important, and it is often the focus of my articles.

What is Oxalic Acid?

Q: *I've been reading your newsletter for a while, and I find it very interesting every time. I find myself eating a lot more raw greens lately, but then arose again a concern that I had when I was full on raw, oxalic acid. Can you help de-mystify this substance? For example, what does it do if taken in too much? How it affects our system?*

I read that it is found in green, leafy vegetables, like kale, collards, and chards and that it can be detrimental if accumulated in too high concentration; it would precipitate the calcium and become toxic. I'm not too sure what to think, but it would be nice to hear about it in your newsletter.

A: Oxalic acid is a chemical found in many plants. This substance binds with calcium to form calcium oxalate, an insoluble salt. Too much oxalic acid, like in older varieties of spinach, for example, can be detrimental. Here are the greens and vegetables that contain oxalic acid: HIGH OXALIC ACID CONTENT: Lambs-quarters, beet leaves, purslane leaves, older varieties of spinach, swiss chard (leaves & stalks), rhubarb, parsley, amaranth leaves, and sorrel. LOW OXALIC ACID CONTENT: Dandelion greens, most fruits, kale, watercress, escarole, mustard greens, turnip greens, kale, broccoli, tomatoes, asparagus, cabbage, and most greens not mentioned.

Anything high in oxalic acid should not be consumed every day or along with other greens high in oxalic acid. Enjoy a wide variety of greens and use tender lettuces as your main greens for salads.

Problems with Fructose ✳

Q: *From reading your e-zine, it seems that you advocate a fairly high-fruit intake, as a way of meeting caloric needs without consuming large quantities of fat. There seems to be a lot of information "out there" these days from other reputable health professionals that discuss the unsuitability of fructose* (i.e. fruit sugar) for human consumption. Their consensus seems to be that consuming fructose is very hard on the liver, that it is immediately converted to fat, and that, overtime, will lead to the condition known as fatty liver. These health people specify that no more than 2 pieces of fruit should be eaten per day as eating fruit, in addition to readily converting to fat, will also cause insulin levels to spike, leading to a whole host of other problems associated with unbalanced hormones. How would you respond to this issue?

A: I really question the "reputability" of the authors who claim that fructose, as it occurs naturally in fruit, could cause health problems, when these authors recommend cheese and red meat that they sell on their websites. In many articles published on Mercola's website (one of the most popular websites on alternative health), the studies cited on the "harms" of fructose were done using refined fructose, such as in the form of high-fructose corn syrup. Mercola incorrectly applies the same conclusions to the fructose naturally occurring in fruit.

Show me just ONE study that proves that eating whole fresh fruits will be detrimental for health, and I will pay attention. Eating a low-fat, high-fruit diet will not cause insulin levels to spike, will not cause unneeded weight gain, and will not cause a fatty liver. People condemning a fruit-based diet have obviously no experience with it at all.

Problems with Low-Fat Diets

Q: I have a question for you. I really like your advice, and it makes a lot of sense. However, every time that I try to go on a low-fat, raw food diet, I feel like I'm going to go crazy. I've been on a raw food diet for about a year, and I feel great almost all the time. I'd say that 90% of my caloric intake comes from fat and protein. The last time I tried to go on an all fruit diet, I stuck with it for a month, eating massive amounts of fruit (at least, way more than I ever have before) and massive amounts of veggies and greens. I started to lose all of my strength, and, after a month, I felt weaker than I ever have in my life (although my body weight remained the same). Additionally, my teeth became really sensitive. I've considered a few possibilities:

1. I did the diet wrong. (I'd think that I should feel pretty good after a month.) Actually, I think this is the best possibility. I tend to do that.

2. You're wrong. A low fat raw food diet isn't the best. People have different metabolic types, and I happen to be one that requires more fat and less fruit.

3. *What actually is happening is that I need more protein or something, for some reason, than some other people, and what my body is screaming at me for is protein, not fat. Maybe I should consider eating something, like spirulina, instead of hemp seeds (a major staple in my current diet, which, by the way, I feel pretty good on).*

Anyway, I was wondering what you had to say about it, because you know a ton more about this than I do, it seems. Thanks a million!

A: Thanks for considering my point of view. I must say that I've tried many times myself to eat a raw, low-fat diet, only to find myself in the following situation:

- The diet fell apart after a few weeks, following a period of extreme cravings for unhealthy foods.

- Out of fear that I was doing something wrong, I gave up completely and did something else.

- I kept trying other diets, which were unsatisfactory; so, eventually, I always found myself wanting to try eating a low-fat, raw diet again.

After these many attempts, I have learned some great lessons. First, now I know that I didn't really know how to do it in the first place! I thought I was doing it the right way, but, in fact, I wasn't. I thought that I had enough information to follow the right diet just because I had read one book on the subject, but, in fact, it wasn't enough information at all! I can't really give you that much information in the context of answering your question here, but I can tell you that:

1) **Chances are great that you didn't do the diet correctly.** Often, just reading a book on the subject isn't enough to get the right kind of knowledge. It usually takes more information as well as actually meeting people who are living this kind of lifestyle who can help to coach you. But, since you haven't given me any information on how you actually did a low-fat, raw diet, I cannot really comment on that.

2) **It's not really about me being right or wrong.** I didn't invent the concept of a low-fat diet. It's what most successful health programs recommend. The concept of eating raw is also one that makes sense, but one thing I know for sure is that the high-fat, raw diet is a recipe for disaster. You get to make your choice between a high-fat and a low-fat diet. Personally, I see absolutely no reason to choose the high-fat diet in view of the predictably bad results it brings and the amount of research that there is to back up the actual dangers of following such a diet.

3) **Metabolic types are a fantasy,** created by those who wish to tell people exactly what they want to hear: "You don't have to change. Just keep on eating the same foods, as long as they're good for your type." If you open a physiology book, you'll understand that the differences in metabolism are very small among people with roughly the same size. Generally, it's less than 5%.

I'm personally someone who's walked around for many years, thinking that because of my particular "metabolic type", I wasn't able to thrive on a low-fat, raw (or mostly raw) diet. I actually started to believe the metabolic typing books, and I did all their tests, only to find out that I needed a high-fat, high-protein diet! This solution proved to be terrible, and the fact is that, once I learned to eat properly, I was able to thrive on a low-fat diet with none of the problems that I had experienced in the past.

4) **Generally, high-protein foods are also high-fat foods.** People who say that they crave protein actually crave calories. It's been found that protein-foods have the highest "satiation" factor, followed closely by carbohydrates. Fats are last on the list; they're the worst. What it means is that if you're deficient in energy intake, you'll start craving all sorts of things, usually proteins or carbohydrates (bread, potatoes, etc.). So it's possible that someone craving proteins is actually not eating enough to meet his/her energy needs. Or, more likely, they are not eating enough of the kinds of foods that will provide enough energy to meet his/her needs. I would like to add that, unless one is experiencing serious growth (teenagers, training bodybuilders, etc.), the protein needs remain relatively the same for each individual of the same size. I highly doubt that someone could need "way more protein" than someone else because of their particular metabolism. It has not been scientifically proven.

Eating Fruit Peels or Not

Q: *Hi! Although our family has been Vita-Mixing for a number of years, we have NOT been doing the 'green' thing, although sprouting has been a minor addition to our food intake. Because of your mega efforts on the raw food movement, we have been enjoying greens more and cooking less! Yeah! And I am a mega, self-taught, gourmet cook!*

A question became apparent recently as to why you suggest eliminating the skins from cucumbers? "Store bought, maybe?" It is my understanding that the majority of vitamins and minerals are just under the skin and since I grow my own in an organic style garden, what is your perspective regarding the skins? Are they toxic?

A: A lot of people will tell you that you need to consume all skins of all fruits, because that's where the "nutrients" are. Those people have not understood the basics of nutrition and the fact that deficiencies are not caused by a "lack", but more often by an "excess", of something.

I've heard people say that the skins of apples are more nutritious than the apple itself. Of course, they were selling a specific supplement made from apple skins.

If the solution were to eat the most nutritious foods to be healthy, then why not eat banana peels? They contain plenty of nutrients.

Fruit peels are not "toxic" but are generally not digested. Even tomato and grape skins just pass through the stools undigested.

So, my point is that there's no reason that should stop you from peeling certain vegetables or fruits. I personally peel cucumbers with thick skins, but I eat the skins from very soft cucumbers, like the English variety.

I eat some fruits with peels, but I do not eat them for the nutrients. I eat them because it's more convenient or tasty to do so.

If I blend something, I will generally add the whole fruit if the peel is edible, but I generally avoid very tough skins, like most regular cucumber skins and mango peels.

I also peel apples when the skin is too tough or waxed. Even though that skin is rich in nutrients, those nutrients are generally not accessible.

Primates in the wild will peel skins of all fruits, and only consume the fruit flesh, unless they are very hungry and, therefore, non-discriminating.

Bottom line: don't try to seek the most concentrated source of nutrients, instead, seek the most absorbable source of nutrients in a food that's easy to digest.

Is the Good Stuff in the Peel?

Q: You say that we should peel commercial fruits and vegetables. However, it is widely and repeatedly reported that most of the beneficial, natural stuff in fruits and veggies reside in the *peel* and surface. So wouldn't peeling your fruit, veggies, etc. greatly reduce the benefits that they would give you?

A: It's a misconception to think that everything that goes in our mouths is assimilated. Nutritionists have a very linear way of thinking. Their scientists analyze foods in laboratories and say: Oranges have more Vitamin C. Therefore, eat more oranges. The peel of fruits has more vitamins. Therefore, eat more of the peel! They forget that the peel of fruits is indigestible. It clearly goes out almost intact in the stools. All of the fruit-eating animals in nature peel their fruits. Monkeys will even peel grapes! But, of course, no one taught them nutrition. The flesh of the fruit is the part that we're supposed to eat, not the peel. If the peel contains tons of pesticides, will you eat it nonetheless just for the vitamins it may contain, that you might not even digest anyway? Many poisonous plants contain lots of vitamins. You could pretty much take any living plant on the face of the earth and find some useful vitamin in them! But the point is that we should be eating the foods that give us the most with the least expenditure of energy. More isn't always more in a good way.

What Raw Foods Should We Avoid?

Q: *I love your website and your videos. I have not seen any reference to raw eggplant: Some websites say it is edible while others say it is not. What is your opinion? Are there other veggies or fruits that should not be eaten raw? Thank you for your time.*

A: Rather than making up rules about what can and cannot be eaten raw, I'd rather have you trust your taste buds. I don't see anything wrong with raw eggplant, except for the fact that it's not very tasty. In the past I have marinated it for some recipes, but I don't think that I've eaten raw eggplant in the past 5 or 6 years!

A few comments about some fruits and vegetables:

Raw legumes (even soaked or sprouted) should be avoided due to the toxic enzyme inhibitors found in them, as well as high quantities of raw starch. Beans should never be eaten raw.

Potatoes and other very starchy vegetables should also never be eaten raw.

Buckwheat greens should be avoided in large quantities due to a substance contained in them called fagopyrin, which can cause hypersensitivity to sunlight.

Rhubarb is a vegetable to avoid because of the high concentration of oxalic acid.

I recommend moderation with any strong or bitter-tasting greens, such as dandelion, watercress, culinary herbs, etc.

It's a misconception to think that everything that goes in our mouths is assimilated. Nutritionists have a very linear way of thinking. Their scientists analyze foods in laboratories and say: Oranges have more Vitamin C. Therefore, eat more oranges. The peel of fruits has more vitamins. Therefore, eat more of the peel! They forget that the peel of fruits is indigestible. It clearly goes out almost intact in the stools. All of the fruit-eating animals in nature peel their fruits. Monkeys will even peel grapes! But, of course, no one taught them nutrition. The flesh of the fruit is the part that we're supposed to eat, not the peel. If the peel contains tons of pesticides, will you eat it nonetheless just for the vitamins it may contain, that you might not even digest anyway? Many poisonous plants contain lots of vitamins. You could pretty much take any living plant on the face of the earth and find some useful vitamin in them! But the point is that we should be eating the foods that give us the most with the least expenditure of energy. More isn't always more in a good way.

What Raw Foods Should We Avoid?

I love your website and your videos. I have not seen any reference to raw eggplant: Some websites say it is edible while others say it is not. What is your opinion? Are there other veggies or fruits that should not be eaten raw? Thank you for your time.

Rather than making up rules about what can and cannot be eaten raw, I'd rather have you trust your taste buds. I don't see anything wrong with raw eggplant, except for the fact that it's not very tasty. In the past I have marinated it for some recipes, but I don't think that I've eaten raw eggplant in the past 5 or 6 years!

A few comments about some fruits and vegetables:

Raw legumes (even soaked or sprouted) should be avoided due to the toxic enzyme inhibitors found in them, as well as high quantities of raw starch. Beans should never be eaten raw.

Potatoes and other very starchy vegetables should also never be eaten raw.

Buckwheat greens should be avoided in large quantities due to a substance contained in them called fagopyrin, which can cause hypersensitivity to sunlight.

Rhubarb is a vegetable to avoid because of the high concentration of oxalic acid.

I recommend moderation with any strong or bitter-tasting greens, such as dandelion, watercress, culinary herbs, etc.

Here are other foods that are not lethal or toxic. These can be considered "borderline", but they might be used as a seasoning:

- **Garlic:** Due to the Allyl methyl sulfide produced from the digestion of garlic and the way it is exuded from the skin pores, causing bad breath and smell, I personally prefer to avoid it!

- **Onion family:** Quite strong and best used in moderation, or oxidized by chopping them in a food processor and leaving at room temperature for a few minutes for the strong oil to partially evaporate.

- **Hot Peppers:** The substance that causes the heat sensation in hot peppers is called "capsaicin". It binds with pain receptors that are responsible for sensing heat. So it "tricks" the brain into thinking that it's sensing heat or pain. The physiological response is the same as when an actual burn has occurred, even though the tissues have not been harmed. Heart rate is raised and perspiration is increased, with the release of endorphins. Hot peppers are a stimulant. Knowing that, I still personally enjoy a little "heat" sometimes as a seasoning.

- **Mushrooms:** Many types of mushrooms are toxic. The cultivated varieties are relatively safe, but I wouldn't class them in the same category as fruits and vegetables. I rarely enjoy them raw, but, sometimes, I might eat them in a recipe.

There are no reasons to avoid any common fruits sold at the supermarket.

Raw Cacao

 Q: *What do you think of raw cacao?*

A: I often get asked what I think of the whole "raw cacao" craze. If you don't know about this, there are some people who currently claim that raw chocolate is the ultimate food of mankind or the "gods" and that we should eat as much as possible to benefit from the high levels of antioxidants, magnesium, and other trace minerals.

Truth is, their claims are completely flawed and wrong. But, it doesn't mean that you have to stop eating chocolate altogether.

Let's take an honest look at the issue, by looking at some claims made about cacao:

"Cornell University food scientists found that cocoa powder has nearly twice the antioxidants of red wine and up to three times what is found in green tea."

Yes, cacao contains lots of antioxidants. But the question is not, "What is the highest source of antioxidants?" but, rather, "What is the "healthiest source of antioxidants?"

Cacao is rich in fat and contains some caffeine and theobromine, which is a stimulant like caffeine. Therefore, one should not eat too much of it.

However, blueberries and other berries are free of these concerns and also contain lots of antioxidants. In my opinion, they are a much *healthier* source of antioxidants.

"As we have noted, cacao is one of nature's richest sources of magnesium, which is a heart, as well as a brain, mineral."

Same here. Cacao may be rich in magnesium, but that's not a reason good enough to make it a main part of your diet, especially when it's rich in fat! Other foods contain lots of magnesium, including green vegetables.

"Cacao, because it is unadulterated, has an even stronger love energy. In ancient Aztec wedding ceremonies, the bride and groom would exchange 5 cacao beans with each other."

What can I say here except that I'm surprised people buy this kind of nonsense. Lots of very unhealthy foods have been praised throughout the world for their "magical" qualities; it's not surprising to find cacao among them.

The bottom line about raw cacao and raw chocolate is that it's not the healthiest source of antioxidants or nutrients, and it's not a "magical" food.

Just like alcohol, tobacco, and drugs, cacao contains stimulants, and it shouldn't be consumed strictly for the health benefits of antioxidants and trace minerals.

I'm all for enjoying food and life and having some cacao as part of your diet occasionally. Enjoying some health benefits that way is perfectly fine. But to make raw cacao an important part of your diet, as is recommended by some people, is completely ridiculous and unhealthy.

Also, most cacao is not even raw; it is processed. If you're interested in raw food and antioxidants, stick to dark greens, vegetables, and fruits, like berries.

Cacao vs. Carob

 What do you think of carob?

 Very few people know much about cacao, where it comes from, and what it actually is in nature.

The cacao tree is a small evergreen tree that grows mainly in Mexico, South America, and the West Indies. The tree bears a fruit that has a white, sweet pulp, containing a number of reddish-brown seeds that are about 1 inch long. These seeds are what are referred to as raw cacao beans. If the seeds are dried, roasted, and then ground, you end up with cocoa, the basic ingredient in chocolate. However, it's the raw and dried cacao seeds that some of the raw-foodists are touting these days.

If you want to get technical, the name of the plant is Theobroma cacao, and theobromine is a chemical related to caffeine. So, even though the raw seeds or ground cacao made into a drink are not as strong as coffee, it's still a stimulant. And it's very bitter.

As I've said before, cacao beans are not really food. If you found them in nature, you wouldn't eat the seeds. You would suck on the juicy pulp around the seeds and throw away the seeds themselves. (In fact, that's how the fruit is sold in the tropics.)

Even if you wanted to eat the seeds, they would not taste like chocolate or anywhere close. In order for the cacao seeds to taste like chocolate and become the cacao beans that we know, they have to be fermented and processed first.

Cacao contains theobromine, which is a stimulant that acts like caffeine. So that's why a 2-ounce piece of chocolate has the stimulating power of one cup of espresso coffee! The same goes for "raw" chocolate.

Now, I know that there are all kinds of good stuff in it, like magnesium and that sort of thing. But you could say the same of all kinds of poisonous plants. In fact, if we could eat them without getting sick, tobacco leaves would probably be considered a "super-food"!

Just because it has some "super-nutrition" doesn't mean it's healthy. A lot of good things have been said about red wine, or even beer, but it won't change the fact that it's an alcoholic beverage. Alcohol is bad for the body. Period.

Raw cacao beans, or "nibs" as they're sometimes called, are now being sold at exorbitant prices by different raw food companies as the latest "superfood" by saying that they have magical properties. I still disagree. First of all, as I said, they are bitter, indicating the presence of a poison. And, when I say a "poison", I'm not making this up. Theobromine may act as a diuretic, too. Additionally, much of the supply of these raw beans is found to have microbe contamination!

Now, I'm not going to say that I haven't tried it and even used it for fun, very sparingly, in some recipes. However, I've never considered it to be a health food. Even though some will say that cacao contains many chemicals that enhance physical and mental well-being, such as magnesium, calcium, zinc, iron, copper, and potassium and that it contains a lot of antioxidants, there are still healthier, safer ways to get these minerals and benefits.

That's why I still prefer to use carob powder in my recipes. Carob powder is made from the pods of carob trees. There are hundreds of varieties of these trees growing all over the world, including the United States. However, the evergreen type in Mediterranean countries produces the most flavorful product and provides much of the commercial carob products.

The pods of these trees are harvested, and then the pulp of the seedcases is broken into pieces called "kibbles". The kibbles are roasted and finely ground. It is naturally sweet and reminds me of chocolate. Instead of being a stimulant, carob is a mineral rich food that has a calming effect. Carob is high in fiber and rich in polyphenols that have strong antiviral and antiseptic properties, making it effective when given to treat bacterial-induced diarrhea.

Carob is a wonderful substitute for cocoa, because it contains fewer calories, is naturally sweet, and, unlike cocoa or sweet chocolate, is caffeine-free. It is non-addictive and has no theobromine or oxalic acid. In addition, it is usually cheaper. It's also low in fat and sodium, calcium-rich, and a good source of potassium. Unlike cacao and chocolate, it does not interfere with the body's ability to assimilate calcium. Now, carob truly is a health food!

Coconut Oil

Given the recent hype, what do you think about the health benefits of coconut oil?

Coconut oil is a concentrated, saturated fat. I've known a few people who got into trouble (liver problems, mainly) by over-consuming coconut oil. Coconut oil is a refined food, like refined sugar. It is pure, concentrated fat. Most people already eat too much fat in the first place, so I don't see the benefits in adding
a concentrated fat like processed coconut oil to their diet.

Also, how do they get coconut oil out of the coconut meat? It has to be separated somehow, and, most commonly, it is done by boiling and scraping the oil off the top. So I really question any of these companies that claim that they have raw coconut oil.

In any case, it still has to be highly processed to get oil out of the meat. Even if you can get fresh coconut oil (like I can in Costa Rica), the people will tell you to keep it in the fridge or it will go rancid in a few weeks. How can all of this coconut oil in health food stores sit there for months and months on the shelf, be raw, and NOT go rancid? If you want to benefit from the nutrients in coconuts, do not consume the oil. Instead, consume WHOLE coconuts, young if possible. You'll get a food that is much more beneficial, much easier to digest, and cheaper too.

Remember, eating whole foods is best. You have all the nutrients in the proper ratio.

Coconut Oil & Omega-3 oils

Q: *You claim that you have done well by eating lots of fruit, as long as you were not also eating lots of fat. It was eating too much fat that caused problems for you. Could you please clarify what type of fat you were eating, and what symptoms showed up when you ate too much of it?*

Did you try switching to another type of fat? I am fond of coconut oil, and I would like to know if you have had problems with it. If so, please elaborate. Have you tried any of the high Omega-3 oils, such as flax oil? Thanks.

A: First of all, I would like to clarify that this claim is actually not "my" claim and not related to my particular experience only. The effects of a high-fat diet are well researched, by many doctors as well.

However, as far as my own personal experience is concerned, I haven't noticed any difference whether the fat came from natural or unnatural sources. Of course, there are other negative effects from eating cooked fats, but you can't logically come to the conclusion that just because it's a "raw" fat that it's okay. It's refined and 100% pure fat. It is highly unnatural to consume it in that state, regardless of the content of omega-3s.

I wouldn't eat coconut oil by itself under any circumstance, but I love to use it externally on the skin and hair.

Additionally, there is no need to consume a special oil to get omega-3 fatty acids. The only reason why people think that they need so much omega-3 is to balance out the excess omega-6 that they are consuming in all the plant oils and animal products they eat. By going on a low-fat diet, you won't have this problem and can get the proper ratio from whole fruits, vegetables, as well as in some nuts and seeds. They have the perfect ratio for you.

Enzymes & Fermented Vegetables

Q: *Fred, thanks for addressing the Kimchee issue. I still have an idea that the fermented veggies are good for you due to the readily available enzymes that are said by some authorities to actually replenish your enzymes bank that depletes with age. I make kitchen with no salt (use culture granules from wildernessfamily. com), a little red pepper only, and with garlic, bok choy, cabbage, a few onions, and NO FISH. It's good actually. I use it for enzyme value and the vitamins and minerals readily available for absorption, as a side dish to some meals. You may want to look at the enzyme issue. The lack of enzyme activity in the body seems to be a major aging factor. It may even relate to Alzheimer's.*

I'd like to correct a few things that you've mentioned:

The whole "enzyme bank" thing is a complete myth. Enzymes are produced by the body when needed, just like hormones are. You are not born with a definite number of enzymes. You can produce enzymes all your life as long as you are healthy. Enzymes in foods are NOT used by the body for its metabolic activities. Enzymes in food are destroyed in the stomach. Raw foods are good for you, but it's not because of enzymes. Another error: "lack of enzyme activity in the body seems to be a major aging factor". A symptom is not the cause of another. Lack of enzyme activity is a symptom that health is failing, but it is not the cause of aging or ill health. If you do enjoy your home-made, salt-free kimchee, then enjoy it. Eat it for taste, not for the enzymes.

Kimchee

Q: *What do you think of kimchee? Koreans eat hot red pepper in their kimchee all the time with every meal. They seem to be real healthy hearty people and their food is applauded as healthy. What do you think?*

A: I do not recommend kimchee. For one thing, it is very high in sodium. Then, it contains hot peppers, which I do not recommend either. Kimchee is fermented, and, in the fermentation process, several vinegar-like acids are produced.

Although they supposedly have some benefits, they interfere with digestion greatly. Kimchee is also seasoned with fish oil. (It looks and smells like a bunch of vegetables that sat in a dumpster for too long.)

I certainly have had my share of kimchee at some point during my raw experiment, but I never felt good after eating it. It is habit-forming because of the high amounts of salt, spices, and vinegar it contains.

I don't think the Korean diet is benefited by the consumption of kimchee. Korean people are relatively healthy (compared to other nations) in spite of the kimchee that they eat, not because of it.

Flax Seed Oil & Phytoestrogen

 I have been taking flax seed oil for some time. I am a male, and I was wondering, since it is so high in phytoestrogen, could this mess with a male's fertility?

A: As you may know, I don't recommend taking flax seed oil or ANY other type of oil for that matter as a supplement. Oil is a refined food, similar to white sugar or white flour.

It's also a highly concentrated fat. It is better to get your essential fatty acids from fruits and vegetables and to only eat limited quantities of overt fats like avocados.

There could be other problems that could develop by consuming this oil regularly, such as the one that you allude to. However, based on the evidence, I don't think flax oil can cause fertility problems.

Goji Berries

Q: *I have always admired your straightforward honesty regarding issues pertaining to the raw food movement and have a few questions to pose to you:*

What is your opinion on raw goji berry powder? I found this product online, and I opted to use this vs. the dried fruit, because I found that the dried fruit too rough on my teeth. Is this an okay product? I'd like to hear your opinion on goji berries, in general, as again they call it a "super" food.

A: Regarding raw goji berries (or goji juice for that matter), my opinion is that this dried berry is rather good as far as dried fruits go. However, again, like every other "super-food" the benefits are exaggerated to make sales. Back when it first came out, I was laughing pretty hard because they were selling it for $35 a pound while you could go to any Asian market and get goji berries for less than $4 a pound. Sure, they were not organic, but the price difference was NOT justified.

As far as the powder is concerned, it sounds like a scam to me. I don't see why anyone would want to order dried fruit powder, no matter how "nutritious" the food is. Sure, goji berries can be a fine dried fruit, but don't spend all of your money on this kind of stuff. This is not going to make any difference to your overall health. Instead, buy good, quality fresh, organic fruits and vegetables, and you'll have a better return for your money.

Greens, Vitamin D, and Bee Pollen

 Q: *I have some questions that don't need really long explanations.*
1. How much is enough greens?
2. What about Vitamin D supplements if Full Spectrum Lighting isn't an option?
3. What do you think about Bee Pollen?

Thank you so much for your time.

A: About greens, we go into more details in the Green for Life Program that I offer online. Basically, 1-2 pounds of greens per day is about what we need. But, then, if they are blended, they are much easier to assimilate, so, in that case, we might need less.

About vitamin D supplements, they might be necessary if you don't get any form of sunlight for months at a time. The best way to check if you're deficient is to get a blood test for vitamin D done and then use a supplement if needed.

About bee pollen, I'm not against the consumption of fresh bee pollen. I have eaten it before and liked it. It's not as sweet as honey, and it is very delicious. However, the dried bee pollen supplements sold in the store as a "superfood" have very little value as they are dried and processed.

Green Powder

 Q: *What of green powder?*

A: Almost every supplement company has a variation of the "green powder", which is basically a powder made with dried grass, dried grass juices, dried vegetables, and possibly algae. This powder is supposed to make your body more alkaline and give you nutrition that you can't find elsewhere.

First, I would say that grass powder is not a worthy food, and anyone that is growing grass, turning it into a powder, and making a lot of money selling it is really laughing their way to the bank at the expense of their unknowing customers. Even if it's called "wheatgrass", it's still grass.

A powder of vegetables or algae can never compare in nutritional value to fresh vegetables, even if those vegetables are not organic.

The real superfoods are dark green vegetables, such as spinach, romaine lettuce, black kale, parsley, celery, arugula, and so on.

With the use of "green smoothies" made with *fresh* green vegetables and fruit, anyone can obtain superior nutrition in a few minutes a day (ruling out the argument that people don't have "time" to eat well).

Green smoothies and fresh raw greens literally put these green powders to shame. For a free mini-course on the power of green smoothies, go to:

http://www.greenforlifeprogram.com

Honey and Molasses

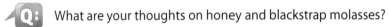 What are your thoughts on honey and blackstrap molasses?

About honey, many people believe that honey has certain healing qualities. Personally, I find it too concentrated to be eaten as a food. It's a concentrated sweet, and it's acidic. Those are two qualities that certainly won't help your dental health. I find honey to be so sweet now that I don't eat it very often. I occasionally use it as a sweetener for a recipe but not by itself. At this point, I prefer to get the natural sugar from fruit instead. About blackstrap molasses, it's true that it's very rich in minerals. But you've got to understand where these minerals come from. They result from the residues of lime and what's left of sugar cane after it's been boiled for many hours at a very high temperature. Molasses is a byproduct of the sugar industry. They used to throw it away, but now it's being sold as a health food.

Noni Juice

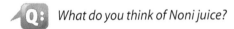 *What do you think of Noni juice?*

Although this discussion could lead me to cover any possible supplement or superfood among the thousands of products available, I think you're starting to get my point.

I'll just finish with an example of a "superfood" called noni and sold as "noni juice".

The noni is a fruit that's been used for centuries in Polynesia for its alleged medicinal properties. However, there is very limited scientific evidence to support these properties.

When I visited Tahiti in 2006, I was on the tiny island of Huahine. There, I had the chance to try real noni juice from a local Tahitian couple who made the juice from their own fruit tree.

Let me tell you, it was the most disgusting, horrible concoction that I ever had in my entire life!

Obviously, the noni is not a natural food for humans, as there is no way anyone would want to consume it unless they thought it had some medicinal value.

My Tahitian friends explained how they prepare the noni juice. They put all these unappetizing, weird-smelling noni fruits in a jar and then let them ferment for several days.

Then the fermented juice that oozes out of the fruits and reeks, like the juice that forms at the bottom of a trash container, is what they drink.

Now American companies have had the great idea of adding a bunch of sugar to this awful tasting Tahitian folk remedy juice, making up a fantastic story around it, throwing in some questionable science, and selling millions of dollars worth of the stuff to gullible people.

Listen closely: it's completely absurd to think that one food can be a universal remedy for all of our ailments. We need nutrients from different sources, and Nature isn't so capricious as to put everything in one place.

We're meant to eat fresh fruits and vegetables, drink pure water, and have a healthy lifestyle with lots of exercise, healthy relationships, and positive thoughts. All the rest is marketing and hype.

Of course, you are free to believe what you want about noni juice and other kinds of superfoods available on the market. But do yourself a favor and make the decision to try for yourself what the study and experience of natural hygiene and health through a pure raw-based diet can do for you.

More on Noni Juice

Q: *I don't know what your qualifications are to rubbish such products as green superfoods and tahitian noni juice, but you have clearly not researched, in any significant way, the Tahitian Noni company in Utah who have spent millions of dollars on noni research and are the largest private company in the world!!*

I personally know dozens, if not hundreds, of people who have benefitted dramatically from the use of their products. Even a peremptory investigation would have shown you that they don't sell pure noni juice as their proprietary blend has been shown to be more effective. (It does not have an unpleasant taste.)

They do not make claims (Other than improved energy and support for the immune system)! I run a health store, and I have no time for the many companies who have sprung out of nowhere making claims for their grossly inferior products. In my store, I have seen dramatic improvements in the health of my clients using green foods in pill or powder form.

I agree entirely about the use of fresh green foods, etc., etc., but obtaining high quality organic foods of this type is not easy or affordable for many people and many simply do not have time (or inclination) to do the preparation.

I feel that you should do diligent research rather than telling your own subjective story about the juice. If you looked into the eyes and spoke to many of my clients about their use of green foods, noni, aloe vera and similar nutrients, you WOULD HAVE DIFFERENT OPINIONS.

Just in case you think that I am in this for the money, I work 7 days, every week, do not have holidays, have not seen my doctor since 1977, am vegan in excellent health (61 years old) and could make more money as a cab driver working half the hours. Bet you don't post this email!!!

Very Sincerely

Derek Rogers

A: I am not against getting different points of view. But, first of all, let me say that, indeed, my blog and website represents MY opinion, and I'm not saying that I hold the ultimate truth. However, I observe certain trends and bring my bit of wisdom to it based on my 14 years of experience in the Natural Health Movement and my study of natural hygiene.

The trend that I have observed is seeing thousands of companies making outrageous claims for an EXTREMELY overpriced product. I've talked about many of these products before, such as goji berry juice and mangosteen juice, just to name a few.

Of course, for each product, there are champions promoting it, lots of supporters for it, and, of course, a hefty pile of testimonials. And they will also all say, like you, that all of the other products are inferior products, but somehow theirs is better.

If noni juice is working for you, then that's perfect. If you find it worth your money, then sure, continue using it.

But, if you say that my experience is entirely subjective, well, I would argue that it is based on a careful thought process. I would rather say that the experience of people experiencing good results from these products is rather subjective.

There are many ways to explain the benefits that someone may get from a particular product, such as noni juice:

- Placebo effect (which is scientifically proven to "cure" 40% of diseases)

- Product forces you to eat less food (either by reducing appetite or replacing meals), therefore benefits are obtained through food reduction

- Product recommendations include other healthful practices, such as exercise and proper diet

- Product contains certain nutrients that may be lacking in a person's nutrition, but that could be obtained at a much lower cost (with homemade green smoothies, for example).

And so on and so forth.

But, for readers who would like to look more into the topic of noni juice and why I'm not the only one to think it is a scam, I offer the following resources:

http://www.livescience.com/health/061017_bad_juice.html

http://noni.worldwidewarning.net/index.php

http://www.bellaonline.com/articles/art4883.asp

http://quackfiles.blogspot.com/2005/07/tahitian-noni-juice-scam.html

Mangosteen Juice

 What do you think of Mangosteen juice?

I'd like to get a few things off my chest that have been bothering me for a while, namely the greed and abuse of consumers credibility of many companies that are selling outrageously expensive products for their so-called "antioxidant" power.

I'm going to first crush a few obvious "scam" products, not because those are necessarily the worst ones out there, but simply because these products get pitched all the time. I know that a lot of honest health-seekers are wasting a lot of their hard-earned cash on them.

Then, after I'm done with this rampage, I'm going to give a last uppercut to these greedy empires by showing you some of the best antioxidant packed foods that you can incorporate into your diet inexpensively.

Xango Juice: The Art of Abusing Credulity

A long time ago (over 16 years), I briefly attempted to succeed in the "network marketing" world. For almost a year, I was involved in one such company, selling "premium dog food", believe it or not!

So I received a lot of insights into the world of "network marketing". While it's certain that there are many good companies that operate under this model, there are definitely a whole lot of bad ones.

When I first joined this MLM (Multi-Level Network) company, the big guru told us that MLM was the future of the world. He also said that in ten years, 80% of the products would be distributed that way (which obviously hasn't happened, 10 years later… not even close). Additionally, he shared that because MLM by-passes the "big distribution network", it allowed the distribution of higher quality products at a lower cost.

My experience with many Multi-Level-Networking companies that I have encountered proves this to be wrong. Generally, the products they sell are very high-priced. Unless you actually join as a distributor, you literally pay several times the actual market value of the product.

I've also found that, while there are a few good MLM companies with good products, most companies are selling suspect items to gullible consumers. Many of these products have actually very little value, and are 90% hype, marketing, and exaggerated claims.

Of course, they always have a cute little story to back it up, like how the founder of the company had a "vision" and a "dream" to improve the nutrition of the entire world, and how he founded his company to fulfill his higher mission.

I, particularly, like how they talk about this one "scientist" from Japan (ever noticed they're all from Japan?) who found the fountain of youth in some ancient plant, and he now wants to share it with the western world.

Let's talk about this Mangosteen Juice.

The company Xango sells their exotic fruit drink made with "mangosteen". This fruit is not related to the mango. When I was in Bali, I ate mangosteens by the kilo, and they were very inexpensive. In Asia, the mangosteen is regarded to be the "queen of the fruit" for its delicate taste.

Xango sells their mangosteen juice as a "miracle cure". Actually, what they sell is some mangosteen product mixed with the juices of about eight other fruits. And at $32.50 per bottle, this fruit juice better be good!

Actually, if you start to believe their marketing literature, this juice is nothing short of a miracle cure. According to Xango, there are more than 20 "human health benefits" to their mangosteen juice, from "anti-microbial" to "anti-cancer".

Supposedly, we should drink their juices because of "xanthones", a "powerful antioxidant" that "may help maintain intestinal health, strengthen the immune system, neutralize free radicals, help support cartilage and joint function, and promote a healthy, seasonal respiratory system".

However, since they don't have any serious research to back this claim up, Xango adds this disclaimer as a footnote: "These statements have not been evaluated by the FDA. This product is not intended to diagnose, treat, cure, or prevent any disease".

Xango is in the business for the bucks.

Anyone who knows network marketing knows how the system works. Independent distributors are selling the products, but mainly recruiting other distributors, in order to get a percentage of their sales.

Generally, the motivated network marketer will aggressively sell the products to his own friends, relatives, and neighbors.

(I remember when I was in this "dog food" company, and I phoned the entire list of names from my high school year in order to pitch them the dog food product!)

With this system, the more distributors a person can recruit, the more money they can make. And the company itself provides all of the marketing material that they need to generate as much buzz as possible.

Like all similar products sold through the same kind of system, Xango has some kind of resemblance of scientific truth that they exaggerate to the extreme to sell their product.

Many of their claims are completely exaggerated and unsubstantiated.
For a neutral perspective on Xango, read the Wikipedia page on the subject:

http://en.wikipedia.org/wiki/XanGo

Countless Other Products

The marketing, the claims, and the suspicious research behind Xango's success mysteriously resembles a lot of other similar products that we've seen marketed over the last few years. I'm referring to:

- Noni fruit juice

- Goji Berry juice -Aloe Vera juice

- Monavie juice

It's the same story here, the same scam, with a different product. In fact, I've found that both the Chief Financial Officer AND the President of Xango worked previously for Tahitian Noni International, another company selling their own miracle cure.

When I look at a $35 bottle of "antioxidant-rich", mangosteen juice, I can't help but laugh and think to myself, "What kind of an idiot would spend that kind of money (plus shipping) for a bottle of fruit juice?"

Let's not forget what these companies are after.

A few years ago, more than one person wanted to take advantage of my "big mailing list" to sign me up as a Xango distributor. They tried to convince me that I would make "so much money" if I used the power of my mailing list to sell this product and recruit other distributors.

I didn't consider it for a single second, and I never replied to those requests (one came from a friend of mine).

What's interesting is that everyone, who came to me to tell me about mangosteen juice, spent more time trying to explain how much money I could make with it, rather than trying to convince me that it was a really good product. It's almost as if the product is irrelevant as long as the rest is in place.

Some Anti-Oxidant Rich Foods: Cheap Alternatives

Okay, now that I feel a little better to have expressed the truth about this mangosteen juice, let me give you some quick tips that these companies certainly don't want you to know.

1- Berries — Berries are by far the one of the richest sources of antioxidants, particularly wild blueberries. I suggest having as many berries as you can in your diet. Plus, they are particularly enjoyable to eat. When wild blueberries are in season, freeze them in ridiculous quantities and use them throughout the year.

2- Pomegranate Juice — Pomegranate Juice is a very high source of cancer-fighting antioxidants. You can either purchase fresh pomegranates and make the juice yourself, or purchase pomegranate concentrate (which is still a high source of antioxidants). The good thing is that even a big jug of pomegranate juice will only cost you about $7, so 5 times less than the mangosteen juice (which is made mostly with other juices). And, best of all, you can find it in most health food stores.

3- Prunes — According to recent studies, prunes rank really high on the "anti-oxidant" score (http://www.webmd.com/diet/guide/20061101/antioxidants-found-unexpected-foods). That's a good thing, because they are also very delicious.

4- Greens — Dark green, leafy vegetables are also an excellent source of anti-oxidants, but it's not only that. Greens contain more nutrition than any other food! For the full story, sign up for the Green for Life Program at http://www.fredericpatenaude.com/greenforlife.html.

5- Mangosteen — Finally, you can also get the health benefits of mangosteen by trying them out fresh. They are very delicious. You can find them in many Asian markets. Even at $5 a pound, you're still going to get a better deal than you would get on the Xango juice. And, if you ever travel to Costa Rica in September or Asia in the winter, you'll get all of the mangosteens that you can possibly eat, at dirt-cheap prices.

Olive Oil

Q: *Why do you say that extra virgin olive oil is not healthy?*

A: I would say that olive oil is not a "health food" the same way that whole foods, such as fruits, vegetables, and avocados are. Olive oil is a refined food. They make olive oil by pressing the olive and throwing the pulp out (with all the vitamins and minerals it contains), until what's left is pure fat. Olive oil is liquid fat. Now, I'm not against using some olive oil occasionally, but I'm simply pointing out that it is not a whole food, and it is not a health food. It's just fat. And, generally, people need to eat less fat, not more. So by cutting out the olive oil from their diet and getting their fat from the much more natural sources of fat, such as nuts and seeds, people will end up in a much better place. Better nutrition equals less fat intake.   In the Perfect Health Program, Dr. Doug Graham and I go into detail about why there are so many things, like olive oil, that are labeled as "health food" but are not.

Protein Powder

 What do you think of protein powder?

Another all-time favorite of supplement companies is protein powder, in all its forms. There's the ultra-refined soy protein powder, whey protein, rice protein, and now a less refined hemp protein.

But the idea is the same: Somehow, no matter how much food you eat, there's still a chance that you might not get enough protein. Therefore, you should consume protein in a concentrated, powdered form.

This idea is especially popular among body-builders and gym-goers. It's interesting to note that starting from the Greek gymnasiums, two and a half thousand years ago, through the ages of gladiators and modern gymnastics, men and women of all ages have been able to build magnificent, muscular bodies by eating nothing more than simple foods and without the use of protein powders.

This is a classic example of how you can market a product by first "creating a problem" that doesn't exist.

Nutrition textbooks teach that you can get all the protein you need as long as you consume enough calories from whole foods, even if all you eat is fruits and vegetables.

Wheatgrass and Spirulina Pills

Q: *Do we need to take wheatgrass pills or spirulina pills? These are supposedly not supplements.*

A: There is very little value in taking powdered grass or powdered algae. First of all, we cannot digest grass very well, even wheatgrass, even when it's dried and turned into a powder. There are also problems associated with spirulina. It contains a vitamin B-12 analog that actually can precipitate a deficiency problem. In addition to that, these green powders are not actually that rich in minerals when compared to the price of greens and vegetables. When you eat plenty of fruits and vegetables, as well as green smoothies, you will be taking in plenty of vitamins and minerals, much more than what is found in these so-called "super-foods".

Chapter 3:
Raw Foods & Health

Can the raw food diet improve your health? Can you or your loved ones be "cured" by raw foods? Are there some specific foods that you should eat for specific illnesses?

I often get these questions.

People are often surprised to hear that I do not actually believe in raw foods. I do not think that raw foods are "healing" or that they have special powers. I also do not think that there are specific foods that should be eaten for specific illnesses.

I believe in the scientifically-proven healing powers of the body.

Whether it is to recover from a cold or to heal injuries, we've all noticed the incredible healing powers of the body.

A healthy lifestyle and a raw food diet can certainly help to assist the natural healing power of the body, but alone they have no magical power of their own.

The most effective, natural cure is actually the simple removal of the cause.

If smoking is at the root of your health problems, the road to recovery starts by quitting smoking.

If lack of sleep and stress is causing your health to deteriorate, fixing those areas are a first priority, and no drug or even natural food will ever substitute the removal of the cause.

If poor dietary choices are the basis of your health problems, then eating a properly balanced, low-fat, raw diet will certainly eliminate almost all of the possible bad dietary choices that could be at cause.

In this chapter, let's take a look at different aspects of raw foods and health.

How to Become Alkaline

Q: *How do I alkalize my body system? What green powder is best to mix with water and drink daily? Is there anything else that you'd recommend?*

A: The best way to get a more alkaline body is to consume fresh fruits, vegetables, green smoothies, etc., on a regular basis. Foods like meat, dairy, grains, beans, nuts, and seeds are considered acid-forming. Reduce or cut out these foods and increase your intake of fresh produce. Your body will do the rest.

I don't recommend any type of green powder. Fresh foods are far better than refined foods for nutrients. Fresh greens in green smoothies would be the best way to increase greens on a regular basis to your diet.

Green Smoothies

Q: *I am SO enjoying my green smoothies. They are great in that now I am eating entire kale leaves, instead of just the juice. My current favorite is 5 kale leaves, 2 pears, and maybe a few strawberries. It feels very nutritious to me, and I thank you for giving me a new way to eat healthier. When trying to eat correctly and lightly (not overloading the body with food), it seems difficult to get everything in. The smoothies seem to be one good answer. One question: are grapefruits all right with greens? I didn't see any recipes with them. I love grapefruit, and I would like to use them more.*

A: Grapefruits are perfect with greens, but I prefer sweeter fruits myself. You should be able to find a few recipes for green smoothies with grapefruit. Try using a sweeter variety, like pink grapefruit, or try just eating the grapefruit by itself. There is no reason to avoid them. They are delicious.

What Body Fat is Too Low?

Your diet recommendations have helped me so much (in a fairly short time), compared to all the other raw food diets. I completed the ten day cleanse program, and I feel much better.

Before the cleanse, I weighed 159 pounds with 9.8 percent body fat on a 5' 10" frame. Now I weigh 153 pounds with 6.7 percent body fat, and a body mass index of 22.1. Do you think 6.7 percent body fat is too low (especially in the winter)?

Also, if I stay on the cleanse diet long term, with 2 ounces of nuts per day, will I gain the 6 pounds back that I lost? Maybe I should just accept the fact that I am slim, since I feel good and healthy at this weight.

I used to eat too many fatty foods to gain weight, but then felt more tired. I think that I looked better when I weighed more, but I feel much better now. I have additional questions below.

Do fruits and vegetables lose much vitamin or mineral content when they are frozen?

Why do you eat so many bananas per day? What is their benefit?

How long do I wait to eat nuts or fat foods after eating fruit?

A: Right now you are at a very enviable spot at 5'10", 153 pounds and 6.7% body fat. I know a lot of guys (including me) who would love to be at that level! So I would not change anything there. Remember that you're still at a very healthy level for a man. If you want more body mass you could add some weight training to gain muscle if you feel you look too thin, but go by how healthy you feel, not just what you think you should look like.

Between 6 and 9% body fat is considered very healthy for athletic men.

But women need a higher body fat of at least 11% to maintain proper hormonal function (hormones are stored in the fat cells). Between 11% and 20% is the ideal range for an athletic woman.

Your body fat and weight ratio indicates that you must be very muscular. You should not have any problems in the winter at all. Just keep up your fitness program and eat sufficient calories.

I have no idea why you would want to gain weight at this point, except to gain even more muscle through your exercise program. Many actors actually train to be exactly where you are so that they can look at their best in a movie!

To answer your other questions: Some vitamins are lost when you freeze foods but not a great amount. Minerals stay intact. I'm not against frozen foods as long as they are not eaten super cold. What I'll generally do during the winter is add a handful of frozen berries to every smoothie. Since the rest of the smoothie is warm or room temperature, it doesn't really taste "cold". You don't want to put very cold foods in your system because:

Firstly, they will make you feel very cold, which is probably not what you want during the winter!

Secondly, too many cold foods can affect your intestinal flora and impair your ability to produce and absorb vitamin B12.

As for the banana thing, I don't think I eat "so many bananas". I eat the right amount based on what I need. There are also many days when I don't eat any bananas at all. But bananas are easy to eat, non-acidic, rich in calories, and fairly inexpensive, so they are the perfect staple on the raw food diet.

Blending and Health

Q: *I thought that blending fruits and greens affected the nutrients inside of them. Is this not the case? Being able to eat them in blended meals would be a dream (alleviate the time-related difficulties of all that chewing). Are we sacrificing any of the vitamins and minerals?*

A: There is some oxidation happening when you blend, so there is a minimal vitamin loss (but no mineral loss). However, many nutrients are made more available in the process, because the foods have been broken down in small particles. So I think it's a good trade-off.

Your food becomes more oxidized the longer you blend as well. So, if you are just blending a simple smoothie or green soup in 20 to 30 seconds, you shouldn't have any major nutritional losses.

Candida

Q: *I was recently diagnosed with candida albicans, and I was told to eliminate fruit for at least 3 weeks. Then, I can add less sweet fruits back slowly. What is your experience with candida albicans? What would you recommend since I was depending on the fruit for calories? I've already lost 15 pounds and only weigh 100 pounds since starting the raw foods diet. Thanks for answering my questions. I truly appreciate your teaching and cookbook products.*

A: I get that question a lot, so I've decided to answer it in a 20-page report on the Fruit Controversy at:
http://www.fredericpatenaude.com/fruitreport.pdf

The fact is, fruit sugar is not the problem with Candida; the problem is when you are trapping sugar in the blood stream by eating fat first or with sugar, which slows down the absorption of sugar by your cells and feeds the candida organism instead.

I'd suggest eliminating fat for 3-10 days and just eating fruits, vegetables, and greens. You will find your candida issues become non-existent and your health greatly improves.

Plus, this is a much shorter trial than trying to sustain on raw food without eating fruit for 3 weeks.

Colonics and Enemas

Q: What is your opinion on colon hydrotherapy and enemas? Some raw-foodists say that these are necessary in the beginning to speed up detox, some say they are necessary for life, and some say they can actually be harmful.

A: I've never recommended enemas and colonics, and I believe them to be completely useless for achieving perfect health. I think that they are actually harmful to your body. We had an entire teleconference on that subject during the "Perfect Health Program" with Dr. Doug Graham, which is available for download or on CD. Hydrotherapy cannot help detoxification, which is a process that occurs at a cellular level. All it does is evacuate the contents of only a part of our intestinal tract (the colon) in a way that is completely unnatural and disruptive to true health.

Also, forcing liquids back up your colon and intestinal tract is seriously invasive and can do more harm than good. You're putting bacteria from your colon back into your intestinal tract where they don't belong, and toxic matter can be reabsorbed through the tissue and actually enter the blood stream. This is a serious risk.

Many people that regularly have colonics have damaged their internal healthy flora in their intestines and become constipated, thus relying on colonics to expel bowel movements for them.

Detoxification is a misunderstood topic. There are no specific foods or procedures that will "detox" the body. It's a process that only the body can do when placed under the right circumstances. Remove the toxins from your diet and lifestyle, and the body will continue the process.

Getting Enough Calories

Q: *I have an important question for you. First, though, you need to know that I am trying to transition to a raw food lifestyle. I am 6' tall and weigh 125 pounds. The problem that I am experiencing is that I eat lots of low-calorie, low-density fruit that fills my small stomach easily and quickly. I want to keep eating to satisfy my hunger, but I can't because my stomach is full. I tried the 7 banana + water smoothie and got sick because I overate, which is very easy thing for me to do! Over eating is one of the biggest problems I have right now. Do you have an answer for this? Any help you can give me will be greatly appreciated!*

A: I suggest eating 5-6 smaller meals instead. Don't force yourself to eat more than you can. Instead, eat more often. With time, you'll find that you'll be able to make your meals larger and accommodate a more optimal volume of food that can provide enough calories to meet your needs.

What you can do now is just evaluate how many calories that you need approximately, and spread that over 5-6 meals, rather having big meals that don't digest properly and slow you down.

Healing Colitis or Crohn's

Q: *Will you please address, particularly for someone like myself, who is just examining a raw food diet, if and how moving to a raw diet may help heal an ulcer and/or diseases like ulcerative colitis or Crohn's?*

A: I highly recommend consulting with David Klein, who's the world's expert on healing Crohn's or ulcerative colitis with raw foods. His website is: http://www.colitis-crohns.com/

Many people have healed and improved their digestion on a low-fat, raw food diet of whole fruits and vegetables. Good luck!

Eating for an Exam

Q: *I have a question: I intend on taking a graduate school exam (MCAT) soon. I was told to eat protein mixed with carbohydrates for energy (since the test is 5 1/2 hours). I was wondering if fruit would work to eat in the morning of the exam, as it may induce me to running to the bathroom. This could mess up concentration as the test is time sensitive. I was wondering if you had any tips on raw foods that I could eat in the morning on the day of my exam that would not induce me to running to the bathroom consistently.*

A: I would be tempted to recommend fasting, although for such a long test it might not be a good idea if you've never done it before. I imagine that the average person doing this test must at least drink something during the duration of the test? The best choice if you want to get mental energy during the test is eating fruit. However, you don't have to eat large quantities, which like you said, might necessitate a few trips to the bathroom. Just a few pieces of fruit, consumed at regular intervals during the test, will give you the energy that you need. Bananas and dried fruit at that time would be a good choice (even though I don't usually recommend dried fruit). This would prevent you from having to go to the bathroom so many times.

Enemas

Q: *I read your book The Raw Secrets. It contains great information that makes a lot of sense! I noticed that you didn't mention enemas. Was this not recommended? After reading some of your stuff, I am left a little confused about enemas.*

A: I haven't done any enemas, even during my fast, and it wasn't recommended in my book either. For a better understanding, read "Fasting Can Save Your Life" by Herbert Shelton.

Enemas and colonics are not a part of Natural Hygiene, and I do not believe they are necessary for good health.

Essential Fatty Acids

Q: *This is actually in reference to your book The Raw Secrets. You said that fats shouldn't be eaten as much and that we should be careful of them. My question is: What about all these essential fatty acids (EFA) that the raw and vegan diets are missing. There is the Omega 3's, 6's, and 9's. I know some of them we need to get from outside sources. What do you think is the best way to get all of these?*

A: In raw, mostly raw, or vegan diets, there are no missing EFAs. In a healthy person, the short-chain, fatty acids are created from other EFAs found in food. There is no need for taking fish oil, EFA supplements, etc. That conversion may be compromised in an unhealthy person. In that case, the solution is not to supplement with EFAs but to correct the cause, which is the wrong mode of living and diet, and improve absorption.

In a fruit/vegetables-based diet, you'll find sufficient quantities of EFAs. If you add in a few walnuts, seeds, etc., you'll get all of the EFAs that you possibly need. I do not recommend any type of oil or EFA supplement.

Quoting Dr. McDougall:

"In man, pure deficiency of EFA has been studied mostly in persons fed intravenously. However, sensitive tests have found deficiencies in elderly patients, people with fat malabsorption diseases, and after serious accidents or burns. EFA deficiency does not occur in people following low-fat diets, because these diets are high in vegetable foods, rich in EFA."

Exercises You Can Do At Your Desk

 I work behind a desk all day. I love my job, but I feel so stiff and out of shape by the end of the day. What can I do to offset sitting for 8 hours a day?

 I've got some great exercises that you can do right at your desk that will have you feeling better and staying more flexible. So there should be no excuses!

Now, here's my 3-part daily plan for you:

1. Stand up!

At least every hour, you should at least just stand up. Reach your arms in the air and get on your tippy toes, trying to elongate yourself as much as possible. Then, come back down on flat feet and reach your right arm up as high as possible, slowly bending over to your left side. Come back up straight, and then reach your left arm up as high as possible, slowly bending to the right side. Shake everything out, and slowly bend forward, letting your arms dangle down. Don't worry about keeping your knees straight or being able to touch the floor. That will come with time. Just use this time to get the blood flowing. Be sure you're letting your neck relax and hang loose. Shake your head "yes" and "no" and let it release. Slowly, come back up to a standing position.

Do this at least once every hour. It does not take a lot of time, and you will soon feel much better.

2. Relax your neck.

Those of you working at a desk all day, probably on the computer most of the time, hold a lot of tension in your neck. It's really important to try to ease that tightness.

First, while working, try hard to keep your shoulders down and your back straight (good posture does wonders for easing tensions and also for good digestion). Be sure your chair is at the right height so that you can comfortably have your feet flat on the floor and your arms are parallel to your keyboard.

Here's an exercise specifically for your neck:

Either standing or sitting, drape your right arm over your head and touch your left ear. Slowly lean your head towards your right shoulder. Be sure that your left arm is held straight down (after a while, you might want to flex your left hand, so that your palm is parallel with the floor for an added stretch). Hold and slowly count to 10. Now, do the other side. Slowly and gently, roll your head clockwise one or two times; then, roll it the other direction.

Try to do this at least 2 or 3 times a day, especially after being at the computer for an extended period of time.

3. Stretch and flex your arms and hands.

Another danger of sitting and typing too much is carpal tunnel syndrome, an ailment where you start to feel pain in your wrists. With carpal tunnel syndrome, you may also experience numbness in different parts of your hands. Anyone who does repetitive motions for long periods of time needs to be very careful about this.

Here are some exercises that you can do to ease the effects of too much typing or writing:

First, hold your arms out parallel to the floor, with your palms facing the ground. Flex your hands up, as though you're about to push against the wall in front of you. Hold, while counting to 10 (for an added stretch, you might want to use one hand to push the other hand back towards you, and switch sides, but be very gentle and don't yank or push too hard). Now, point your hands and fingers down towards the ground (again, you might want to very gently push the opposite hand toward you for more stretch). Now, hold your arms out to your sides and repeat the hand stretches up and down. Push outwards with your arms. Now, raise them up and interlock your fingers, facing your palms towards the ceiling. Push upwards, try to reach and push the ceiling. Bring your arms down and shake them out. Make fists with your hands. Then stretch out your hands and fingers and wiggle them.

See, that didn't take very long either.

Try to be more aware of sitting for long periods of time. Get up and do these simple exercises. Or go for a walk down the hall and get a glass of water (you can never drink too much water!). Walk up and down the hallways for 10 minutes, then get back to work. You'll feel better and, ultimately, you'll be more productive in the work that you do!

Fasting

Q: *Thanks for your e-zine, I really enjoy the publication. It is really insightful and very inspirational. I am confused about your previous fast though. My question is related to fat reserves. You say that the body lives on its own fat reserves during this period. But, what if you don't have much fat on your body to begin with? Being a raw-foodist in itself makes your body lean, the very food we eat is free from fats that we would store. Wouldn't your own body then start eating away at the next available source of energy, being your muscles, in which the heart happens to be one? This sounds dangerous! I can't wait to hear your answer. I know you have one for me.*

A: That's a good question. Even a "skinny" person still has fat reserves, although not as visible as the average person. Fat is always right underneath the skin and lining the internal organs. Don't forget that the body can convert carbohydrates into fat for storage; it just takes more energy to do so. So you don't need to eat only concentrated fatty foods in order to have body fat. The body only consumes about 1 pound of fat per week, on average, during a fast. The rest of the weight loss is actually water loss. In my own case, my body fat level was quite low before the fast (around 8%). After 23 days of fasting, I was down to about 4% body fat, and I still had some to go! It would have taken another 2-3 weeks to get me down to zero. So, as you can see, even a thin person has enough reserves to fast 3-4 weeks, under proper supervision, of course.

Short Fasts

Q: *I have recently become interested in partaking in a fast. I have read your article about your 23-day experience and find that simply amazing. However, I do not intend to attempt such a great feat right away, although I do wish to accomplish a small 3- to 5-day fast. I was hoping that you could provide me with the necessary information to complete this goal as safely as possible. Thank you for your time and consideration.*

A: As mentioned in my books, it is not safe to fast more than 3-5 days on your own. Do not attempt such a fast on your own, even if your initial experiment seems positive or easy. A short fast can be safely undergone on your own, but, if you have any health condition, you should consult a qualified health professional before attempting it. It is important to know that the "real" fast doesn't really start until day 3, or even day 5-6. What does that mean? During the first days of the fast, your body lives on its immediate reserves: the glycogen stored in the muscle, the food still in the digestive tract, etc. Then it slowly goes into the fat-burning metabolism where it starts to burn its fat reserves as fuel. However, it is still beneficial to fast only a few days (1-2), just to give the digestive system a break. Ideally, you want to rest as much as possible. Plan to spend all day in bed. If you fast a few days but work all the time because "you have so much energy", the benefits of this fast are very limited. It is better to fast 3 days in bed than 10 days while working. This way, you will lose minimal muscle mass as your body isn't converting it into fuel to sustain you. You also want to drink enough water so that you go to the bathroom 6-8 times in 24 hours. Also be aware that during a fast, even a short one, you can get dizzy quickly when standing up, can pass out, and may hurt yourself. So it is imperative that you move slowly when getting up. If someone around you is not supportive of you fasting, it would be a bad idea to attempt a fast on your own.

Health Tests for Effective Raw Food Eating

Q: *Thank you for the excellent article and focus on raw food strategy. In regards to health tests, such as blood work or anything else, what do you recommend?*

I searched the web to come up with effective health testing. I finally found something that made sense to me, but, when I came back to order it later, the website was gone.

Life Extension Foundation did an article on Carol Alt. In the article, it stated that health testing (no specific tests mentioned, I believe) was part of her health management to make raw food eating effective. Thanks for your time.

A: There is no reason to order any health tests from any website unless you absolutely need to know something specific in order to make an important decision about your health. All of these so-called tests are nothing but marketing schemes.

Also, using blood tests to evaluate your health will generally be misleading because you're comparing yourself to an average of unhealthy individuals, which comprises most of the population and are the standard for these tests. This could give you many false positives and negatives and be inconclusive for any deficiencies that you may think that you have.

I'd suggest getting a test done with a natural health practitioner or someone with experience with raw vegan diets. This should be someone who would be able to guide you in determining any deficiencies or problems with the results of your blood test.

How to Deal With the Gnawing Sensation

Q: *I am trying to eat meals only when I am truly hungry. Do you have any tips on how to ignore the gnawing in my stomach? As I understand, the stomach growling, or empty stomach, does not necessarily mean you are hungry.*

Of course, I'm used to eating the second my stomach is empty. Is there a way that I can make the gnawing sensation go away, like drink water? It's very difficult trying to focus at work/studying when my body is doing this!

A: The answer is to learn to simplify your meals in order to ease your digestion so that you get less of the growling on an empty stomach. What I've found is that by eating a low-fat diet with proper food combining, I can easily go several hours without eating without getting much "dissatisfaction" from my stomach. Often, when I run errands, I won't eat before 1 or 2 in the afternoon.

Make sure that you are eating enough calories. You don't want to feel dissatisfied and constantly hungry all day either. You can try drinking water to see if you're truly hungry still. True hunger is a feeling in the throat though and does not come from the stomach.

Hunger

Q: *I recently purchased and read **The Raw Secrets**, and I just have a couple of questions about hunger. One, I understand the difference now between true and false hunger, but, if the symptoms of false hunger are not hunger, what is my body trying to tell me when I experience those symptoms?*

Two, if one is above their ideal weight, is it possible or likely that if they eat only when hungry, they will consume few calories because their body won't signal hunger very often until they have reached their optimal weight?

And my third question is this: I have been trying to eat a 90-100% raw food diet, and I have been only combining foods that combine well. Yet, if I eat only when hungry, I only consume about 750 calories in a day. What is the cause of this, and what should I do about it?

A: 1) Generally, the symptoms of false hunger occur as a consequence of wrong eating habits. Stomach rumblings, heartburn, and appetite are not true hunger.

2) Yes, if one needs to lose weight, their body will not manifest true hunger as often.

3) It's important to eat when hungry, but it doesn't mean that you have to wait until you are *ravenously* hungry. I want to avoid being negative here, but I think the idea is more to NOT eat when you are NOT hungry, rather than only eat when you are *extremely* hungry.

Also, it is essential to engage in some form of physical activity during the day in order to "earn your food" and create true hunger.

Make sure that you eat enough to sustain yourself. I don't know how long you could go eating only 750 calories a day and maintaining your lifestyle.

Not Thriving On Raw

Q: *I have been studying raw-foodism for some time, and I have moved in that direction significantly over the past few months. I would like to make the transfer to 100% raw, but I run into situations that I need to solve for myself.*

I can eat a balanced raw food diet for 3 to 4 days, and then, at about 6 in the evening of the last day, I will get the "gnaws" for something. I will try an avocado, some raw muesli, or some almonds, trying to understand what that grinding restlessness is.

Typically, I my meal plan looks like this:

7:00 a.m. - Diced apple and 1/3 cup of muesli (sunflower seeds, flax seeds, almonds, raisins, and oat bran)

9:00 a.m. - 1 Grapefruit

12:00 p.m. - Fruit salad of tomato, avocado, cucumber, Greek olives, and dulse

3:00 p.m. - Sun tea (peppermint)

5:00 p.m. - Green salad, black olives, cauliflower, leaf lettuce, cucumber, with balsamic vinegar and olive oil.

By 6:00 p.m., I sometimes get the "gnawing". It's not hunger, because I feel full. I just don't feel satisfied. So, I begin this search for satisfaction. If I eventually have an apple fritter or bread, then I am satisfied. However, I feel heavy and have a loss of energy and mental clarity. When it comes, it is strong. Sometimes, I break down and have buttered popcorn with salt, and that doesn't do it either until the bread.

Is this compulsive eating, and I need to work with it that way?

Is it a carb addiction?

Is it an imbalance to my diet even though I have sweet fruit, fatty fruit, and green veggies?

I am willing to face this issue head on. Do I need to walk thru this for a week or a month until this craving is broken? Do I need to juice fast to break through this block? Maybe I need prayer and scripture time to carry me beyond this?

I am just not sure how to approach this challenge. Should I approach it psychologically, physiologically, or spiritually?

Any suggestion to the evening "gnaws" would be helpful. I suspect that grapefruit would suppress this. It's strange to have a full stomach and still be climbing the walls in restlessness for something else.

Any insight you might and could share with me would be helpful. Obviously, being intellectually convinced of this lifestyle is not enough. I want to know how to embrace this without it always being a white-knuckle experience.

 Thank you for writing.

To respond to your questions, let me take some time to analyze your basic raw diet first.

You say that you eat a balanced raw food diet. Well, I've been looking at it, and, to me, it's quite obvious why you have those cravings.

Your basic diet is not something that you can maintain in the long term. You are getting approximately 1000 calories a day, which would be enough for a sedentary 85-year old lady, but probably not for you!

Also, your diet is over 60% fat (by calories), which seriously compromises your nutrition and health potential.

This is not an emotional issue or "carb" addiction. You've simply been eating the wrong raw diet, and, thus, you're body is doing the right thing by "requesting" more sustaining food!

For a start, I would recommend replacing your lunch, which is currently a fatty vegetable salad (with the avocado and olives), by a large fruit meal or several fruit smoothies. Right now, you are seriously under-eating carbohydrates and overeating on fat. You are also under-eating in general.

Also, your breakfast contains a little fruit (apples) and mostly fat (nuts seeds) in total calories. I'd suggest having a large quantity of fruit for breakfast, like 2 melons, 5-6 mangoes, 5-6 bananas, fruit smoothies, etc.

My book, *The Raw Secrets,* contains all the necessary information to get you started with a sustainable raw diet.

Also get educated about calories and start tracking them until you get a good handle on what enough calories for your needs looks like at each meal. There are almost no calories in greens and veggies, so they should not be the main part of your diet. They should be in addition to sufficient quantities of fruit. Eat many pieces of fruit, not just an apple here and grapefruit there.

You could also try "mono mealing" your fruit meals, where you choose 1 fruit and only eat that for a meal like a whole melon, 6 mangoes, 5-7 bananas, a whole papaya, etc.

You're not feeling satisfied until you eat bread because your body needs carbohydrates, and you are simply not providing it with enough. So you end your raw food day with bread instead of eating enough calories from fruit, which is much healthier and easier to digest.

Nutrient Requirements on a Raw Vegan Diet

Q: *I wouldn't have bothered you, but for some time I have been desperate to get an answer to the question of adequate nutrition on the raw food or vegan diet. When discussing nutrients, I need specifics. What are the daily requirements of *essential* amino acids, fatty acids, vitamins, and minerals met on the raw food or vegan diet? Most health authorities that I have encountered agree that a vegan diet is healthy, but only in the short term. Consequently, I am afraid to totally switch over to the diet until I can get some answers. Do you have this information?*

A: Any form of quantification over the exact amount of certain nutrients that we need is totally arbitrary and, at best, very inaccurate. There are so many factors that come into play in determining how much of each nutrient that we need.

Here are some of those factors that influence our needs for specific nutrients:

- Our activity level
- Age, gender, and height
- Muscular mass
- The intake of other nutrients (everything is co-dependent)
- Sun exposure
- Genetic predispositions

In addition to those, there are "new" nutrients constantly being discovered, so we can only guess that we only know a tiny bit about essential nutrients and their relationships with each other. Therefore, there is most likely a lot of nutrients that you could probably worry about, but we don't even know that they exist yet!

I'm sorry that I can't give you the kind of authoritative answer that you're looking for. Are you saying that you believe that the Standard American Diet gives us adequate nutrition?

If you do believe that when you listen to "most health authorities", then you probably are not looking at the evidence in our society of:

- Rampant obesity

- Rampant diabetes

- Rampant osteoporosis and low-bone density (despite consuming an abundance of calcium)

- Rampant illnesses of all kind

There are hundreds of vegan experts. Some of them have done extensive research to prove that you can get better nutrition from eating plants only. Just read the books of Dr. Fuhrman, Dr. Klaper, Dr. McDougall, and others, and you will be convinced. All of their books are backed up by extensive research.

Unfortunately, this kind of research is not available on the raw vegan diet. However, the raw vegan diet is not that much different from the vegan diet. After all, there are no nutrients found in cooked vegan foods that you can't find in raw vegan foods.

So as long as you understand the principles of optimal vegan nutrition, which include:

- Nutrient density

- Low-fat in the diet

- High carbohydrate and low protein

- Simple food combination

... you will understand that the same principles apply to raw food nutrition. Thousands of people throughout the world are transforming their health by eating more raw foods, and thousands of people every day are dying because of their belief that a Standard American Diet is adequate.

Are you going to wait for approval from experts to do the right thing for you? Do you realize that those experts themselves suffer from innumerable health problems and have misled the American public for years by recommending heavily processed foods?

Potassium Overdose

Q: *A question popped up the other day about potassium intake. With some folks relying so heavily on bananas for the bulk of calories, i.e. eating 10+ a day, is there any risk of potassium overdose? I did a little bit of research on the web, but I could come up with nothing definitive.*

A: There's really no point to fear any potassium "overdose" even when eating a fair number of bananas. Research done on wild monkeys showed that they eat over 6500 milligrams of potassium per day, which would take you over 15 bananas to eat as much potassium as they do. Plus wild monkeys are smaller in size than we are, so we could eat even more bananas and not even reach the potassium intake a monkey has on a daily basis.

Early humans consumed 40 times as much potassium as sodium. It makes sense because we lose potassium a lot faster than sodium.

Even standard nutritionists agree that most people do not eat enough potassium and that ideally they should consume close to 5000 milligrams per day, and even more for active people.

Your body regulates any *excess* potassium for you, so there is no need to worry.

Ripe Fruits and Nutrition

Q: *One thing I wanted to know: what about fruits and vegetables that are not yet ripe? It seems that we cannot purchase any that is actually ripe.*

What is the difference in nutrient content if the produce has to sit on the counter to ripen as opposed to ripening on the tree/vine?

A: Unripe fruits will have fewer vitamins than ripe fruits, but the mineral content will not change as much. Perfectly ripe foods have not only more vitamins, but they are also less acidic/ have more vitality - however you want to define it!

What I choose to do is buy fruits in advance that are not ripe and let them ripen on the counter. Some fruits like pineapple do not ripen further; they are either picked ripe or unripe. In that case, always look at, smell, or touch the fruit to assess its ripeness.

Salt Elimination

Q: *Because of heart problems, it has been recommended that I eliminate salt from my foods. I've been using Bragg's Amino Acid liquid for 3 years. What can replace it with and still get the amino acids?*

A: I applaud you for eliminating salt and "Bragg's Liquid Aminos" from your diet. This product is not only very high in sodium but also artificial. Try looking into how the product is made, and you will find that the information very vague and unconvincing as a "raw" product.

However, I don't understand your concern. Amino acids are part of every living structure. You can get them just by eating any fruit or vegetables. You certainly don't need a product that claims to be a source of them. How do other animals get their amino acids? They don't use any supplements or refined foods to do so.

If you need help replacing the salt, I suggest dehydrating some chopped up celery and turning it into a powder in a coffee grinder. It has a light salty taste, and I haven't noticed any problems from occasional use.

The Big Picture about Salt

Q: *The issue of salt is unsettled for me. Aside from whether this or that salt substitute is good or not (Nama Shoyu, Bragg's, etc.), the question remains whether or not sea salt is any good, that is, if it is usable by the body. You say (I don't recall where) that the body cannot process sodium from a mineral source but only through plants. However, as I hear other views, I'd like to hear something more extensive from you on the subject.*

A: I have studied this topic extensively, because I consider myself excessively drawn to salt since childhood and the bad habits I developed then. However, the issue is very easy to understand:

The problem comes from excess sodium. It doesn't really matter what the source is or whether the body supposedly can or cannot assimilate it.

I have not claimed that sea salt is "unusable" by the body.

The problem is excess.

Our bodies need approximately 500 to 800mg of sodium to function optimally. That's about the amount you would get in a diet of fruits and vegetables with no added salt with enough greens.

You can probably get away with getting about 1000-1500mg of sodium per day. At over 1500mg, you will start developing some health problems in the long run.

At over 2500mg, you are starting to seriously jeopardize your health.

And beyond that, you are almost certain to develop a long-term health issues, such as high blood pressure.

Is it any wonder that 90% of the population suffers from this disease?

Whether you get this sodium from celery or from sea salt, it doesn't really matter. It's sodium.

It's just that it would be very difficult to get this amount of sodium from just eating celery. You would have to eat over 30 *large* stalks of celery to get more than 1500mg of sodium. I don't know about you, but, if I eat around 5 stalks, I've had enough.

And, yes, there's also the consideration that sodium coming from an *organic* source is *probably* a lot better than coming from a rock.

So, in practice, you should avoid added salt. This includes Nama Shoyu, Bragg's, sea salt (ALL kinds), Tamari, Herbamare, etc.

If you sometimes add a bit of something with salt in it (such as seaweed powder or even sea salt), it will not affect you as much, because it's the overall picture that counts — what you do every day.

Salt and Water

 You state that we should not take salt (sea) and not drink water. Are you writing this for SAD or RAW readers?

I never said anywhere that one should not drink water. I simply stated that on a raw food diet it wasn't as necessary to consume AS MUCH water as on a Standard American Diet (SAD). Cooked food, essentially, is dehydrated as most of the water is cooked out of it. It is recommended to drink 8 glasses of water a day to compensate by the severe dehydration that occurs when consuming a high-fat, high-salt, high-refined sugar, and cooked diet. When you are relying on juicy fruits and water rich vegetables for the majority of your hydration, you do not need as much additional water. As for salt, I still maintain that sea salt isn't the best choice for our health. Our sodium requirements are very low and can be met by eating green vegetables. A little seaweed, occasionally, can also be okay. Consuming more sodium than what is necessary can lead to several health problems, including hypertension, osteoporosis, and stomach cancer. It also deadens our taste buds so that it is more difficult to enjoy fruits and vegetables without seasonings. Added sea salt is not necessary for a healthy diet, and it is certainly not a health food in itself.

Can Teeth Be Rebuilt?

A: *Thanks for letting me ask this question that has remained unanswered for years by raw-foodists, and everyone else for that matter. Can the teeth be rebuilt? And, more importantly, if, yes, then how? Several of my teeth have crumbled and fallen out, and a dentist wants to take all of them out because the remaining ones are decayed. I have eaten predominantly raw for over 8 years now, although a lot has centered around nuts and dried fruit, which I can see maybe was a mistake. However, I had no guidance and thought I was doing better than the general population. Anyway, to make a long story short, I need help. Many thanks again for any advice you can offer.*

Q: Your question assumes that raw foods have some kind of magical special power and that they can do anything. Unfortunately, cavities can only be reversed in the very early stages. If your teeth are in that state, there is nothing that will rebuild them except dentistry procedures.

I suggest to everyone, especially on a raw food diet, to stick to a strict dental health regime, brushing, flossing, using an oral irrigator, and getting regular checkups. Dental decay and cavities are caused when the saliva is acidic, and there is food to feed the bacteria in your mouth.

Dried fruits and nuts are some of the worst offenders as they can stick to teeth and cause problems if you do not brush soon afterwards.

Can Raisins Prevent Cavities?

A: *I recently saw an ad for a book where it was mentioned that raisins prevent cavities. So I decided to do a search, and this is what I found. nteresting, indeed.*

Q: That's very misleading information. Raisins, as well as any type of dried foods, can cause cavities, and fast. Just ask any dentist. Raisins will stick to your teeth and feed the greedy bacteria, which, in turn, will produce their acids that will eat away your teeth.

If you eat raisins, make sure that you drink water to rinse your teeth or brush and floss afterwards to prevent any problems.

Stevia and Teeth

A: *I use stevia glycerite to sweeten my tea several times a day. Is that bad for my teeth?*

Q: Stevia is not a sugar, and, therefore, it doesn't contribute to dental problems.

Toothsoap

A: *Is it mainly the glycerin in regular toothpastes that is bad for the teeth? Does that mean I shouldn't use regular toothpastes now and then or alternately?*

Q: Commercial toothpastes as well as natural toothpastes contain lots of ingredients that are unhealthy, such as sodium lauryl sulfate (foaming agent) and fluoride. Teeth are best cleaned with a brush or electric brush and toothsoap. However, even if you use toothsoap, you can use other toothpastes now and then, and I'm sure you will notice the difference.

Vitamin D and Vitamin B12

Q: *What brand/type of sublingual vitamin B12 and Vitamin D do you recommend?*

A: The best brand of vitamin D is exposure to natural sunshine, about 30 minutes per day at mid-day in northern latitudes, and any time except mid-day in the tropics. Some studies say that people in northern latitudes cannot achieve proper vitamin D levels from sun in the fall and winter. If that is the case for you, then you may want to look into some alternative vitamin D supplementation for good health.

For vitamin B12, I still stand by my recommendation. I follow the lead of most vegan doctors who recommend supplementation "just in case". The sub-lingual varieties are best.

Chapter 4:
General Questions about the Raw Lifestyle

There are no universities teaching raw food nutrition, but the basic principles of nutrition taught in textbooks also apply to raw foods. However, a lot of what we've learned over the years about the raw food diet and lifestyle comes from personal experience and trial and error.

There's a lot of confusion in the raw food movement about what to eat. One author says one thing; the next says the complete opposite.

My goal has always been to follow the basic principles of health and always question everything. Don't accept what one author says just because it sounds great. Do you your own research and learn to think for yourself.

In this chapter, I want to share my experiences and save you some time by answering tricky questions about raw food nutrition.

Allergic to Avocados

Q: *I have acquired so much great information and fabulous recipes from your books and e-mails. Thank you! I do have a question: I am allergic to avocados and most of your recipes contain this ingredient. Can you suggest a substitute in your recipes? Thanks.*

A: It would be a bit of an exaggeration to say that "most" of my recipes contain avocado. In any given recipe book, maybe 5 to 10% of the recipes will contain this ingredient.

My suggestion is to use nuts instead. All dressings containing avocado can be made with nuts. The taste won't be the same, of course, but the results will be similar.

You can also make a delicious guacamole using green peas. I included this recipe in my book "Gourmet Raw Food Cuisine", which is now available as a bonus for the Raw Vegan Mentor Club at:
http://www.fredericpatenaude.com/mentorclub.html

Here's the recipe:

Peamoli

2 cups fresh or frozen green peas

2 Tbsp. olive oil

1 lemon, juice of

1 medium garlic clove

1/4 sea salt (optional)

1 tsp. dulse powder (optional)

1/2 cup tomatoes, diced (cherry tomato halves are best)

Blend all ingredients, except the tomatoes, in your Vita-Mix or food processor.

You may also homogenize the peas in a Champion or Green Life juicer with the blank plate on, and add the other ingredients separately in a bowl.

Add diced tomatoes, and then mix well.

If you use frozen peas (organic only), you will have to let them thaw overnight or rinse them under warm water.

Add the dulse powder if you prefer a "smoky" flavor.

Serve with sticks of celery, carrots, peppers, and green vegetables.

Are Cooked Minerals Inorganic?

 There's so much controversy or conflicting info from different sources. It would be helpful to address the following questions in more depth to clarify the issues:

- Do minerals in food that gets cooked turn inorganic?

- Is oxalic acid in raw spinach harmful, or is it harmful in cooked form only?
- You say that sprouts have toxins, and so they should be avoided. On further inquiry, I found that Gabriel Cousens states that the toxin canavanine in alfalfa sprouts is mild, that one would have to eat a lot of it to have toxic effects, and that as it is water soluble, by the seventh day of rinsing, it is mostly gone. Is that accurate?

TC Fry has the philosophical position that anything that Nature intended as food for us would have no toxins, and, thus, he dismisses sprouts. Well, so many vegetables have slight amounts of toxins that we might as well eat next to no vegetables!

I take that as an extreme position. A philosophy is a good rule of thumb, but it can become a dogma (just like, "If it's raw, it's cool!"). These are some ideas to play with. Thanks, and I really do appreciate your approach to diet.

A: To answer your questions:

- Cooking does not render minerals useless in the body. If that were the case, then nobody eating cooked food could stay alive. So the answer is: no.

- That's an interesting question about spinach and oxalic acid. The problem with oxalic acid is that it can combine with calcium to form calcium oxalates. However, what I've found is that the spinach grown today in North America contains much less oxalic acid than in the past. When I travel to other countries where they grow older varieties, I find the spinach impossible to eat raw because of the high amount of oxalic acid. But, if you eat the common "baby spinach," there's nothing to worry about. If it bothers you, reduce the quantity that you are eating.

- Sprouts contain toxins, but, like Gabriel Cousens mentioned, the risks are minimal in small quantities. I'm opposed to buckwheat greens because of a very strong toxin contained in them. Read more about it here: **http://www.gillesarbour.com/buckwheatArticle.php**

In general, you cannot avoid toxins completely in natural foods. But, like you said, the amounts are minimal in vegetables.

How can you tell? If something is palatable to the taste, when eaten raw, without seasonings or combinations, then it's human food.

If it's too strong, too bitter, or otherwise unpalatable, then it contains toxins and should be avoided.

Then, from those general principles, you can make a few exceptions, for example, with mild spices, such as dill, cilantro, green onions, etc.

Are Raw Recipes Healthy?

 In your food combining article, you stated that one should not combine avocados with nuts (so as not to combine two types of fatty foods). I'm perplexed by this because one of the most common raw recipes that I've seen is a nori roll recipe that includes at least three types of nuts and avocado. Are you saying this should be discarded?

 Yes, this food combination is an absolute disaster. Raw recipes are not created by people with any nutritional training. Same goes for gourmet chefs who cook in fine restaurants. Meals are designed for taste and appeal and not for proper digestion and health.

My recommendation would be to avoid these recipes, or simplify them so that you are not regularly consuming multiple types of fat. Certainly, do not eating overt fats more than once a day. Add more veggies and cut out the unnecessary nuts or avocado. You can make many delicious nori rolls with only avocado and veggies or just veggies.

Certain Gurus Look Good or Bad

Why do certain leaders in the raw food movement look bad for their age?

I received some emails about how someone decided to NOT follow the raw diet, because they thought Dr. Graham looked bad.

While others told me that they decided to follow it, because he looked good. Someone else decided NOT to follow the high-fat diet because they thought that David Wolfe looked bad, while Roger Haeske looked better. In the end, people have different perceptions about who looks GOOD and who looks BAD, based on their own criteria.

You shouldn't make it the decisive factor. I prefer to look at a number of people following the same diet, especially if they've been doing it for several years. There are more important factors than just looks. Try to evaluate health as a whole instead. Many people teach about raw food, but they do not get sufficient exercise, sleep, or sunshine. These make a big difference as well.

Cooked Tomato Paste and Lycopene

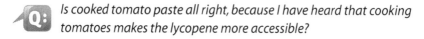

Q: *Is cooked tomato paste all right, because I have heard that cooking tomatoes makes the lycopene more accessible?*

A: Lycopene is just ONE phyto-nutrient, and there are thousands of them in food. It doesn't even make sense to start worrying about all those little phyto-chemicals. Just eat fruits and vegetables, and you will get all the lycopene and other nutrients that your body can use. It doesn't make sense to eat cooked tomato paste (a refined food that comes from the factory) just to try to get an isolated, over-hyped nutrient. Instead, eat whole tomatoes and do not even worry about the lycopene. You are getting plenty. Just watermelon or pink grapefruit alone has more lycopene than tomatoes! You don't hear about them being cooked do you?

Dealing with Mosquitoes

Q: *There are a lot of great hiking trails out here in Ohio, but sometimes the mosquitoes can be a little bothersome. A couple of people have told me that eating a clove of garlic will keep them away (I don't plan on trying this). Are you aware of any better tasting/natural ways to keep the bugs away without turning to repellent? Are they more attracted to you if you eat a lot of fruit?*

A: I haven't found that the mosquitoes are more attracted to fruit eaters, but they seem to be more attracted to certain people! I found citronella essential oil to be excellent for this purpose. You don't have to use the repellent. This essential oil alone gives excellent results.

I have heard that some high fruit eating or fruitarians don't have many problems with mosquitoes, but they claim they did when eating a lot of spices or cooked food. Perhaps mosquitoes are attracted to certain human smells and eating a high-fruit diet with no spices makes you less appealing.

European Units of Measure and Natural Hygiene Books

Q: *I have bought the book **Instant Raw Sensations**, and I really enjoy it. The problem is that I am living in Austria, and we do not use "cups" as units of measurement.*

A: *Also, I am looking for good books about raw food. The problem is that most of the raw food books are very confusing, especially the German speaking ones. **The Raw Secrets** is definitely one of the best books that I have ever read about this topic. Which books from Albert Mosséri and Herbert Shelton (there are quite a lot) would you recommend and are still available?*

1) 1 cup is 236 milliliters. I found this website that does the conversion for you: http://www.easysurf.cc/cnver2.htm#cptoml3

2) The books by Herbert Shelton that I have loved the most and that I recommend to everybody are:

Fasting Can Save Your Life

The Science and Fine Art of Food and Nutrition

Health For The Millions

Natural Hygiene: The Pristine Way of Life

Fasting For Renewal of Life

Food Combining Made Easy

As for Albert Mosséri's book, if you read French, the books are still available directly from him (he's now in his 80s). The ones that I would recommend are:

Confiez Votre Santé à la Nature

Santé Radieuse par le Jeûne

Le Jeûne: Meilleur Remède de la Nature

Mangez Nature, Santé Nature (Tome 1 & 2)

Eating Raw Food Before It's Cooked

Q: *I have a question: I have read somewhere that all raw food should be eaten before any cooked food. Is this correct?*

A: Yes, it's better to eat raw foods before cooked food. This prevents a phenomenon called "digestive leukocytosis," which is the proliferation of white blood cells after the consumption of cooked foods. Also, the principle of "nutrient density" says to consume more nutrient dense foods first. That means raw foods first.

Fred's Fasting Experience

Q: *I am a bit flabbergasted that you did a 23-day fast in Costa Rica. I do agree that perhaps a 3-day fast is healthy, but, beyond that, can't the heart just collapse unexpectedly? How does the doctor explain that danger? I just don't understand why humans have to be so extreme! I'm glad that you are okay!*

A: Fasting under proper supervision is a natural process that most people do not quite understand. The human body has the capacity to live 5-6 weeks without food (or even longer), and at least 3-4 weeks before going into a starvation mode. The difference between starvation and fasting is that, during fasting, the body lives on its body fat reserves, while, during starvation, the body starts to plunder the vital organs of the body to survive. It's a major distinction. I did not fast until starvation, but I still had reserves to keep me going for another week at least.

That being said, I don't recommend that anyone fast without proper supervision. Even short fasts can be a potential health risk if done without supervision. Seek out a licensed professional with a good track record.

What Fred Eats

Q: *What would really help me is to know what you eat, say over 2-3 days, so that I could judge whether what I am doing is similar to what you are. Additionally, it would just be interesting to know.*

Sure, let's see if I can outline that for you. What I eat really depends on what's available and in season. Here's what I ate yesterday:

• Morning: a big fruit soup made with cantaloupe, tangerines, pineapple, and apple

• Noon: I had a smoothie, containing about 6 mangoes and a bunch of purslane (a wild herb)

• A few hours later, I had about 12 red prickly pears.

• Then, dinner was a big salad, containing fresh romaine lettuce, arugula, tomatoes, and a dressing made by blending 2 tomatoes, two handfuls of spinach, and an avocado.

I find that I'm able to have only 2-3 meals a day if I eat enough fruits and vegetables, and especially enough fruits that have high-caloric content, such as bananas, figs, mangoes, persimmon, jackfruit, durian, etc. If I run short of those foods, then I have to eat more often. But I also find that I can easily go several hours, or even a whole day, without eating and without "passing out" or experiencing any other discomfort.

I also love to make raw soups for dinner, and, occasionally, I eat steamed vegetables.

Household Products and Toxicity

Q: *I read your book this weekend (The Raw Secrets). I love it! It answered my questions regarding raw diet. You did mention that household products are not good for you. I have been trying to get information on this subject. Could you tell me where I can get information about the effects of household products, and how I can replace my household products with non-harmful ones? I have been looking, and I can't find anything on this subject.*

A: When I mentioned household products, I was referring to all the detergents, bleach, dishwashing liquid, and other common household products, which all contain strong and toxic ingredients. If you want a complete list of all household products and their possible toxicity, along with alternative products to use, check out the book called The Safe Shopper's Bible.

Over-Consumption of Stevia

Q: *I have stopped drinking diet soda and coffee for several months now by replacing it with drinking a lot of herbal tea with Stevia. The good news is that I am completely off all artificial substances, and I have not touched diet soda or coffee (nor do I want to go back). I thought the Stevia consumption would go down over time. However, it's been several months, and I am still using just as much as I did when I went off the diet soda. I can go through about a 60-ml bottle every 2 weeks. Is this too much? What are the dangers of the over-consumption of Stevia?*

A: Just to clarify for our readers who might not know what stevia is: stevia is a plant bearing green leaves that have the particularity of tasting very sweet without containing any sugar. I've had the occasion to try fresh stevia leaves, and they certainly can be a nice addition to salads, smoothies, and fun to eat plain, too. Stevia extract, on the other hand, is a refined product that comes in two forms: One is a green powder that is made, basically, from the dried leaves of the stevia plants. Another extract is even more refined, and it is sold as a white powder. Stevia extract is also sold in the form of a clear liquid. All of the stevia products mentioned taste extremely sweet; yet they do not contain any sugar. They are certainly much less harmful and more natural than the other artificial, no-calorie sweeteners, such as splenda and aspartame, whose negative health impacts have been demonstrated several times over. That being said, I do not know what the dangers of consuming stevia extract or powder might be. I certainly think that there is always a potential danger in consuming a refined product on a regular basis. Let's not fool ourselves here: stevia extract is an extremely refined product. If the consumption of stevia can help you get rid of the soda habit, it certainly can be a good thing, just like drinking a decaffeinated coffee can be a good thing to help you get rid of the coffee habit. But, eventually, that crutch has to be left behind. Personally, I have a method for getting rid of any sugar addiction that never fails. My method acknowledges the fact that humans have a natural sweet tooth for a reason: we are meant, actually designed, like other primates, to consume natural sugar in the form of fresh fruit. Any refined sugar is going to pose serious health threats, but not the natural sugar in fruit that we are meant to eat. My recommendation is to start eating more fresh fruit. Once you eat enough fresh fruit (which by the way, is probably a lot more than you can imagine right now), it is impossible to crave any concentrated sweets, including:

- Chocolate

- Soda

- Dried fruit

- Pastries

- Even bread and other cooked grains

I encourage you to leave that stevia habit behind. If you want to eat stevia, grow the plant! They actually make nice indoor plants. To get rid of your sugar cravings forever, start eating more fruit and less refined carbohydrates.

Washing Produce

Q: *What do you clean your produce with? Do you do anything special? What is the best, in your opinion, way to clean fruit/veggies?*

A: Good question. I peel what I can and use a special non-toxic soap to clean certain non-organic fruits. This soap can be found in most health food stores. I use it to wash grapes, figs, bell peppers, etc., when they are not organic.

What about the Latest Raw Food Books?

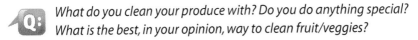

Q: *There's a new book that came out claiming that raw chocolate is the best food. But you say chocolate is "bad, and this book says it is good. I It is the same for lots of other things about raw food nutrition! I believe more in you than in other raw food "gurus" (or the like), but I am extremely confused. I do not know what to think about chocolate and everything else anymore! I really liked your book The Raw Secrets, but then I have wondered what is right to eat, since most recipes contain garlic, onion, oil, and spices. And the more I read, the more I get confused. For example, I tend to refuse to believe that such a millenary food like bread could be harmful for man. What about onion and garlic and the famous Hunza nutrition? You see, I tend to believe in raw food nutrition, but I have lots of doubts, and I wonder if our instinct might be enough for us. You have been very clear and exhaustive in your book, but perhaps you should clarify even more.*

A: Here we go: confusion again!

Someone comes up with a book saying that chocolate is the best thing that you could eat (and they happen to sell it, of course), and then a whole lot of people write me and ask me what I think about it because they get confused. "Could this be true?" But, of course, thousands of diet books are printed every year, and, among them, you'll find an amazing amount of contradicting information. I personally do not have the time (or desire) to go through all of them. And I think it'd be a waste of my time to even try to verify all of the ludicrous statements made by the various authors and self-proclaimed diet gurus. Going back to a natural diet is based on the very simple principles that can be hard to put into practice. In fact, "simple" is harder than "complicated" in this world.

At some point, we have to put some trust in Nature. This year, a book comes out claiming that chocolate or raw cacao is the best thing in the world. Next year, it's going to be something else. Do you have to put to the test all of the sometimes ridiculous theories out there about nutrition and everything else? Do you have to always be in a state of doubt? Remember, success is impossible to the doubter. You have to have a little trust. Only then, success becomes a possibility.

Our natural diet should be composed almost exclusively of fruits and vegetables, eaten as much as possible, in their natural state. You should read again the chapter where I explain the natural law of dietetics or how every creature on this planet selects foods according to three criteria:

*Is the food pleasant to the taste, smell, and sight, when it is consumed in the raw state, without seasonings or combinations?

*This simple test should help you determine which foods are the best. In the meantime, we know that raw cacao is a stimulating and highly addictive food. Humans have done perfectly well all over the planet for hundreds of thousands of years before cacao was discovered, and they were doing much better in every regard before bread and grains were consumed, only thousands of years ago.

Eventually, you will move from trust (which comes from reasoning) to experience. Experience will teach you the principles that you have learned in the right books. For example, you can read my article on raw cacao and still think to yourself, "Yeah, right. I still want to try it." Then, when you spend the night in your bed, restless and unable to sleep, you might think to yourself, "Well, maybe it's true. Raw cacao really is a stimulant."

Or you might read what I have to say about garlic and onions, avoid them for about a month, and then eat some again. Then you might notice how not only your breath has a nasty garlic flavor to it the next day, but also that your fingers, arms, and, actually, every pore of your body has a slight garlic smell. The body is getting rid of the toxic compounds found in garlic!

I, personally, always have to remind myself to put my trust in Nature and to always go back to the basic principles, which are the foundation of any true system. Simple is always the best, but our world responds to "The Next Big Thing" or "Miracle Cure" because we've been conditioned to hype and marketing.

How to Kick the Sugar Habit Forever

Q: *One question I would like to see covered: How can I kick the soda habit? This seems to be a downfall for me. I can be eating great all day, and then, by late afternoon, when I start to wind down, it seems the need for a soda appears. I am down to maybe two a day now, but I still cannot "kick the habit". Do you have any suggestions?*

A: I prefer to look at it from a purely nutritional perspective. What I've found is that once you learn to eat enough fruit to cover your caloric (energy) needs, you simply won't be craving sugar of any kind. Once you eat enough fruit, the desire for cakes, soda, chocolate, and other sweets will have as much appeal to you as a piece of dry cardboard. Even complex carbohydrates (bread, etc.), will have little appeal. Most beginners have no idea how much they need to eat when they switch to a raw diet. Eating 3 or 4 bananas seems like a lot to them, but, in fact, it's not even going to give you 15% of your energy needs for the day. In order to banish cravings for sweets and carbohydrates, you're going to have to eat a lot more fruit than you think right now is a generous amount.

How to Transition

Q: *I'd like to know how to get started. Giving up bread and grains has not been that bad with a filler, like soy, but now that soy is gone, what fillers should I use? Veggies and fruits are good, but people need more. Oh, did I mention that I don't like nuts?*

So what do you do? How long did it take for your mind to settle for less? How did you give up sugar? What are "on the go" meals for you? What fills you up?

A: My cravings are for fruits and vegetables. The trick is to consume enough of them so that you fill all of your nutritional needs, while at the same time avoid the foods that trigger cravings.

You will get "filled up" when you consume enough volume/calories from fruits and vegetables. It's important to understand that those foods are not as dense as bread and meat. You need to eat a lot more of them! It just takes a bit of practice, that's all.

Completely eliminating bread and grains is essential to get your cravings back for fruit. I've noticed that people who eat bread are not attracted to fruit. It's one or the other. Eating both would be too much sugar for the body.

Giving up sugar was one of the easiest things that I've ever done. If you eat enough fruit, you'll completely lose your cravings for ALL artificial sugar, and ALL of the foods that contain them, I guarantee.

Meals on the go are very easy. I prepare fruit salads, smoothies, or salads in advance. Smoothies keep well in a glass jar.

I recommend the following transition, starting from a Standard Diet:

1- Give up junk food: fried food, fast food restaurants, etc. Most people are already at that stage. Start eating more fruits & vegetables — increase raw content by calories.

2- Give up dairy products, especially cheese! Cheese is highly acidic and contains far too much fat.

3- Give up flour, gluten, bread, soy, and sweets. If this is too difficult, use spelt, millet, or buckwheat. Replace sweets with fruit. Progressively decrease the fat content of your diet.

4- Avoid commercial meat and farm-raised fish. Seek wild fish (they are less polluted — see the list), wild game, and free-range eggs. Reduce the consumption of these animal foods to less than 5-10% of your daily calories.

5- Increase further percentage of raw, unprocessed foods, by calories, and reduce salt intake to natural sources and less than 1000mg per day on average. Introduce green smoothies, salads, raw soups, fruit meals, etc.

6- Pay attention to eating when you're actually hungry.

Urine Therapy

Q: *What is it with raw fooders and drinking urine? I don't know what you Canadian and American raw-fooders do, but here in the UK I know of plenty who believe it is healthy and good for our bodies to drink our pee.*

I do not have any inclination to do it, and I think that if my body is getting rid of this stuff then I'd be pretty dumb to override my body's intelligence by putting it back into my body again.

A: You said it right. Personally, I think drinking your own urine is as dumb as hitting your own head with a hammer.

I don't recommend it, and I think eating a healthy diet is far better than drinking your urine for health benefits.

Hot Water and 100% Raw

Q: *I know you believe in limiting eating/drinking ice; what about drinking boiled, hot water? Also just a question about what 100% means. Is eating nori seaweed, carob, agave, and dried fruits 100% raw, or is it just acceptable? Thanks!*

A: I have nothing against drinking hot water, if it's to "warm you up" during the winter. You could even add a little lemon juice. Just be careful not to burn yourself! The lining of your esophagus is very delicate.

As for the other foods that you mentioned, most likely they are not truly raw, but they can still be consumed on occasion. I'm not really a big fan of seaweed, for many reasons, but a little on occasion to make sushi rolls, for example, is okay by me. Agave nectar is a concentrated processed sweetener that I don't recommend either. I prefer to use sweet fruits, such as mangoes, if a recipe calls for agave nectar. I might use honey or dates instead in a recipe if mangoes are not available.

Dried fruits should be avoided most of the time, because they are difficult to digest, tend to ferment, and also stick to the teeth, which can cause dental decay. However, they can be very useful in exceptional circumstances when carrying fresh fruits would be difficult. For example: traveling in the desert, hiking across a national park, visiting remote islands in the South Pacific, etc. Just make sure that you increase your water intake to compensate.

What Is the Best Water?

Q: *I have been studying about different waters. I was told recently that the best water is oxygenated water. What is your opinion and where can I find a machine to make the best water to drink. I've recently moved into a house that was built in the 1830s, and I'm a little leery of the water pipes. The water smells like iron. I really need to find the best solutions.*

A: I'm not so concerned about finding the absolute, ultimate, definitive kind of water. You want to drink pure water, not polluted water. There are many ways to purify water, such as distilling, high-quality filters, reverse-osmosis, and so on. Those are all great ways to obtain pure water. I do not advocate one type of water as being "the best".

Reverse osmosis and distillation are the only ways to completely purify water, but, most of the time, I drink my tap water, which in my house comes from a well and has been tested for purity. I wouldn't do this anywhere else because the quality of tap water in most cities is extremely questionable.

There will always be new ways to purify water, and there will always be people to sell those machines, claiming that their water is "the best". I also think that people in the natural health movement make a much bigger deal about finding the "best water" than it actually needs to be. I suggest that you find a solution that works in your situation, for your budget, and in your home. An Internet search for water purification solutions in your area will be a good start.

For more information on the water debate, please visit my other website **www.waterdebunked.com**

X-ray Machines When Traveling

Q: *The last time I was traveling, I noticed a sign on the carry-on luggage x-ray machine that read: "Caution radiation". I had gorgeous organic orange peppers in my carry-on and immediately became sad upon the realization that my tasty treat was now going to be radiated (similar to microwaved). Do you have any opinion about this?*

A: I'm not too worried about this. Sometimes health food enthusiasts become really worried with all these things that it becomes an obsession. But just flying in an airplane is bad for your health, to some degree, so is watching TV, and working at a computer. I call it a compromise. Maybe some people are going to go live in the woods and try to avoid all of that, but, for me, it's a form of snobbism. You can't escape the age in which you live in. Compromises are unavoidable. That being said, I once carried some seeds through those X-ray machines, and I later tried to sprout them. They did sprout. So I don't think that the machine fries your peppers like a microwave. Don't worry about this and enjoy your trip.

Chapter 5:
Food Combining

Food combining is the concept that certain foods, combined together, are more difficult to digest than if they were combined differently.

When eating raw, food combining rules become less important because there are fewer ways to combine foods together. High-protein foods are difficult to digest when combined with starchy foods, but, fortunately, both of these categories are avoided on the raw food diet.

The main combination to avoid most of the time is concentrated sweets with concentrated fats (for example: almonds and raisins). Unless consumed in small quantities, this combination leads to fermentation and gas.

In this chapter, we explore some questions about food combining and other tips related to optimal digestion on the raw diet.

Digestion Time of Fruit

Q: *I find your ideas concerning raw foods both insightful and similar to my own. I eat mostly fruits (one at a time) and greens throughout the day, but I like to rotate what I eat.*

My doctor told me that you only need 30 minutes to digest between fruits, but the Fruitarian Network says at least 90 min. I was wondering about your outlook on how long to wait. I am especially confused on vegetable-fruits, like tomatoes and bell peppers. I would love your feedback to sort all of this out.

A: I don't think there's a "magic" number for the digestion time of foods. Some people have much stronger digestion than others. I don't suggest eating fruit every 30 minutes or even every hour. Instead, have a meal that will sustain you for a minimum of 3 hours.

So you could eat 1 or 2 kinds of fruits with greens if you were having a large meal or simply fruit alone in a large quantity.

There is no need to wait 30 minutes in between eating each separate kind of fruit. It would be far less tedious to just eat 1 or 2 types of fruits at a time instead.

Tomatoes and bell peppers should digest fine, just like fruits. They're high in water content as well.

Fat Eating Time

Q: *Since you say you should have fat once a day, do you recommend doing so during lunch or during dinner?*

A: I did not say that you should have fat once a day. I said you should not have fat MORE than once a day. The best time will be after you've done your exercise for the day. So for most people that will be for dinner.

You can eat a little bit of fat after your fruit or vegetable soup in a large salad or recipe.

It's best for digestion to not eat fat more than once a day because on a raw food diet you will be eating carbohydrates in the form of fruit for most of your calories.

Food Combining Issues on a Raw Diet

Q: *I'm an actor on CSI and have been moving towards the raw diet slowly over the past year. Regarding raw food combinations, I have experienced some hard core indigestion since I switched to my 80% raw diet. There are occasions when I have consumed a 100% raw diet and end up having some of the worst heartburn and digestion problems that I have ever experienced. Prior to moving towards a ealthier diet, this never happened. Any info on correct food combinations would be appreciated.*

A: First of all, I must say that you've given me very little information to begin with, so my answer will be very generic. Most people who move to a raw diet initially experience some digestive issues as their body is clearing up the old stuff that built up inside of them. This generally lasts a week or two, sometimes 3-4. If it goes on for much longer, there might be something else going on.

But, in addition to that, most people also eat the raw diet without paying attention to food combining and make a lot of other mistakes that make things worse. Maybe you are eating too many acidic foods that are causing you problems, like nuts, seeds, sprouted grains in prepared recipes, etc.

Here are some tips that I can give you for now:

1- Generally, it's better to eat only fruit during the day and vegetables in the evening. Fats, such as avocados or nuts, combine well with vegetables but not with fruits. You can use small amounts of citrus fruits with fats, though, if you need calories.

2- Bananas should not be combined with acid fruits, such as pineapple or oranges.

3- Acid fruits, such as oranges, should not be consumed in excess.

4- Remember to KISS - Keep It Sweet and Simple.

Try looking at what you eat and then seeing how your body reacts to it. Also stay away from raw gourmet meals if you know you have problems digesting them or feel unwell afterwards.

Food Combining Acid with Starch

Q: *Thank you very much for sending this list of food-combining rules, I found it to be very informative. I have been eating raw now for several months, and I feel better than ever. I do have a quick question for you. In your rule #2, you state that we should not combine acid with starch, for example, a tomato sandwich. However, what is your opinion of making a tomato sandwich, where the starch is made from Ezekiel bread? That's become a staple for me: Ezekiel bread/hummus/spinach/tomatoes.*

A: In reality, this is not great food combining. But you're the one to judge. If you get gas, or any other signs that digestion isn't optimal, then I suggest leaving out the tomatoes from that mixture. However the tomatoes are much healthier for you than the bread. You might even find that Ezekiel bread is hard to digest in itself! Personally, I don't really eat any form of sprouted or cooked grains. Grains are just not that appetizing to me or an ideal food. They are acid forming, slow down digestion, and ferment easily in the digestive tract. Look up Grain Damage by Dr. Doug Graham for more information on why grains are so harmful. Also note that there are an increasing number of people who are genetically allergic to the gluten in grains, and this is called Celiac Disease.

You could try making delicious lettuce wraps though and omit the bread altogether. You should have no problem digesting that.

Food Combining and Eating Seeded Grapes

Q: *Maybe I'm being too finicky, but I just wanted to check: Is it OK to eat whole seeded grapes, that is, combining the sweet fruit with the seeds (which I presume are proteins like any seed or nut)? Nature provides them together, but I don't know if that combination is good for humans.*

A: There is no reason to actually eat or chew grape seeds unless they are so small that you can't avoid swallowing them. When you eat seeded grapes you should not chew the seeds so the whole food combining issue at this point is irrelevant. They do not taste very good and can be removed before eating.

Most fruit is eaten without the seeds except for soft easy to digest seeds in cucumbers and the white seeds in watermelon.

Quite often even these seeds pass through you without even being digested. So we weren't meant to be chewing fruit seeds as a staple to our raw food diet.

Green Smoothies and Food Combining

Q: *You talked about food combining and sequential eating as being both good for our digestion and our health. But, for some time, followed by family Boutenko, you have promoted green smoothies as a very healthy kind of food. My question is: Are green smoothies really healthy and not contradictory to the rules of food combining and sequential eating?*

A: Food combining and sequential eating rules go together. Sequential eating is a little more "advanced" (or simple, depending how you look at it...).

My point was that if a food combination can be bad, the sequence in which we eat foods can also be bad, or more optimal.

The combination of green leafy vegetables with fruit is a good one. The sequence of eating fruit and then greens or greens and then fruit is also good. Therefore, it's still a good thing to mix greens and fruit, if you're going to mix anything at all!

Vegetables are different. They do not mix well with fruit as they are often high in starch, but they do mix well with greens. Greens mix well with most things and green smoothies should be no problem to digest.

Lemon and Food Combining

Q: *I have been paying special attention to maximizing my efficiency at following the basic food combining rules that you lay out in The Raw Secrets. I was wondering about combining lemon juice with my salads. Rather than using a homemade raw salad dressing, like I used to do, I have been using the juice of one lemon on my salads to keep my fat intake low. Will the lemon juice react with the greens to cause indigestion? I don't put avocados or nuts/seeds in my salads anymore, because I believe that you said fats before greens, not with the greens. So the lemon juice would only be added to things like cabbage, collards, sunflower sprouts, tomato, celery, romaine, etc. Should there be any concerns with doing that?*

A: To answer your questions, you can certainly add some lemon juice to your salad. It won't cause problems unless you use too much of it, which I doubt you are doing.

I never said to eat fat before greens, but I did say not with greens. Some avocado with a salad is okay. Sometimes, I add a little lime juice on top of it, too, and it digests perfectly fine. The problem is eating a big salad and then eating large amounts of avocado, nuts, or gourmet raw dishes. You would have problems digesting all the different kinds of foods properly and, no doubt, have bloating or gas as well.

Mixing Fruits with Fat

 *In **The Raw Secrets** book it states that we should not mix fruit with fatty foods (like nuts, seeds, or oils) because the fruits may ferment since they digest quicker. So, how long should we wait after eating fatty foods to eat fruit? Is two hours enough time? Thanks.*

A: For the answer to that question, here is the latest article I've written on food combining:

Rethinking Food Combining Rules:

The other day I was eating a delicious salad made with the following ingredients:

- Crisp romaine lettuce

- Sweet and ripe raw corn

- Garden-ripened tomatoes

- Diced mango

- Small amount of avocado

- Fresh herbs picked from the garden

- Lemon juice

I can't express how delicious this salad was. It was truly amazing! And part of the reason why it was so good is because it was made with fresh and ripe ingredients.

But another reason was the combination of the sweetness in the mango and corn, the savory taste of the tomatoes, vegetables, and herbs, combined with the creaminess of the avocado.

I was telling another raw-food friend about this salad, and her reaction was: "Yeah, but what about food combining rules! You say that we should never mix fat with sugar".

Indeed, what about food combining rules?

The raw food diet is a pretty strict diet to begin with.

We don't eat bread. We don't eat meat. We don't eat dairy products. We don't eat eggs (at least most of us don't!), and we don't eat most of what other people eat as well.

But, on top of that, we have these rules about not being able to combine certain foods with each other and how just eating one food at a time is best.

And, I must say, for a long time, I subscribed to all of these rules. But I also knew that not all food combining rules are valid.

For example, the original book Food Combining Made Easy by Dr. Shelton gave a lot of rules with no reasoning at all behind them.

Also, a lot of people have misinterpreted that book. Because Shelton said "eat melons on their own", some people think that they should never eat melons with other fruits (such as peaches), when in fact Shelton clearly stated that you could do so.

Essentially, his rule was meant to avoid the common combination/ abomination in those days of a big slice of watermelon after of rich meal of meat and pasta.

In my book The Raw Secrets, I simplified food combining rules in the raw diet to three essential rules:

- Do not combine fat with sugar

- Do not combine acids with starch

- Do not combine different types of fatty foods within one meal

I'm going to simplify these rules even more, and completely deconstruct the food combining theory!

How I Reconsidered These Rules

For many years, I followed food combining rules blindly without questioning them. Then I started simplifying them over the years, and I realized that some of them weren't necessary.

At this point, I have eliminated most of the "rules" I once thought were essential.

Over the years, I've watched some other raw-foodists eat who didn't know these food combining rules.

One raw-foodist simply made combinations that she liked and that tasted good, without paying too much attention to the combinations, like I did.

My big surprise was to realize that I could eat many combinations that I thought were "bad" without any negative effect whatsoever.

The main combination I'm talking about has to do with mixing fat and sugar together.

Why Certain Combinations Occur in Nature

The idea behind many food combining rules is to simplifying the process of digestion. So, naturally, the "sandwich" is one of the worst combinations ever, because it combines many classes of foods, which are optimally digested in a completely different acidic or non-acidic environment in the stomach.

In the raw food diet, we naturally avoid most of these combinations, leaving mainly one: the combination of fat and sugar.

The idea behind this rule is that combining fat and sugar, such as dates and almonds together, will let the sugar ferment in the stomach.

The reason is simple: almonds and other fats take a lot more time to digest than simple sugars. If you eat them together, the sugar you eat will spend much more time in the stomach and intestines and start to ferment.

But, even with that rule, the traditional rules of food combining allow for certain exceptions. For example, you can combine acid fruits with nuts together.

The idea is that because nuts digest well in an acidic environment, acid fruits don't compromise that picture. They also contain less sugar than other fruits.

This line of reasoning always appeared a little suspicious, but I noticed that the effects of that combination were generally positive, as long as I ate very small amounts of fat.

But here's one strange observation:

- Many foods in nature contain the combination of fat and sugar in significant proportions!

For example, the durian, a beloved fruit of many raw-foodists, is very rich in sugar and quite rich in fat (20% on average).

Even avocados contain some sugar and carbohydrates, and so do nuts.

And surprisingly, all fruits and vegetables contain a certain percentage of fatty acids.

There are also other fruits in nature that contain this forbidden mixture of fat and sugar, such as the "Ackee fruit" that is popular in Jamaica.

So it seems to me a little strange to completely ban this combination, when you can enjoy a ripe durian, which contains a mixture of fat and sugar.

Raw-Foodists Eating Too Much Fat

After thinking about this a lot, I have realized that most raw-foodists who benefit from these food combining rules have something in common: they eat too much fat!

I agree that the combination of a huge handful of almonds with a bag of dates is a nasty mixture that leads to a lot of fermentation and gas.

But, try eating three dates and three almonds together. You'll probably find that this combination goes down perfectly well.

The same goes for other fatty foods:

Eat a huge serving of guacamole and then have all the figs that you can eat, and you probably will experience some gas.

But, if you dice up a third of an avocado in a salad that contains lettuce and mango, you'll probably be fine.

So my main observation with the rule of not combining fruit and fat together has to do with quantities.

When SMALL quantities of fat are used in the diet, there is no reason to fear combining some fruit with some fatty foods once in a while.

So my new "rule" is this: you can throw in some fruit in a salad containing some fat. Try to avoid fruits that are very concentrated in sugar, such as dates, dried fruits, or bananas, and instead use juicy fruits. Also, avoid large quantities of fat.

Eating More Fruit is Better than Eating More Fat

Another problem with the food combining rules that have been presented before are the restrictions that they pose on people.

Let's say you have a salad that contains some avocado.

According to food combining, you should not eat anything for several hours after that, or only eat more of the same ingredients for optimal digestion.

So, if you're not satisfied after a meal of a salad and avocado (and most people aren't because they didn't eat enough fruit during the day or before the meal), your only option is to wait several hours or eat more avocado.

What I recommend now is to eat fruit, whenever you feel like it or feel hungry, even if the combination is not perfect.

Eating some fruit after a salad containing avocado will be a LOT better than eating more avocado and more fat after that same meal.

The Spirit of Food Combining Rules

I still believe in the spirit of food combining rules, which is about keeping things simple and avoiding long lists of ingredients.

However, it's probably not necessary to obsess about these rules, when you can enjoy some simple, tasty, and low-fat combinations that will taste great and digest well, even if they don't follow the rules 100%.

Chapter 6:
Athletes on a Raw Diet

One question that should be asked before evaluating any diet is, "Can it work for athletes?"

Athletes have high nutrient requirements to sustain their amazing performances, so they need to pay attention to their diet. If a particular diet only works for people who are detoxing and want to lose weight, but cannot sustain athletic endeavors, then it is simply not something that is sustainable in the long-run.

Fortunately, a low-fat, raw food diet works extremely well for athletes. In fact, it can dramatically improve their performance.

One important criterion of a diet for athletes is that it must contain enough carbohydrates to fuel the body.

On the raw diet, those carbohydrates can be found in fruit.

One of the many reasons why a high-fat, raw diet doesn't work is because it doesn't contain enough carbohydrates to provide enough fuel for the body. That is why many people are not experiencing the levels of energy that they should when eating this way.

In this chapter, we explore some topics related to not just athletic performance, but health and fitness in general.

Athletic Training and Raw Food

Q: *I have a question regarding athletic training and raw foods. I run and lift weights as my main form of exercise. Should an athlete who is consuming all raw foods simply eat more of what they're eating? Or should they add different types of food to their diet, such as more seeds or greens?*

Sometimes, I wake up around 2:00 a.m. with hunger pangs. My guess is that I'm not getting enough calories, especially on my workout days. My thoughts are that I should just add more quantity of the same foods that I'm already eating. Would more leafy greens and fruits be the way to go? (Twice a day, in the form of salad or raw soup is my favorite way to consume greens.) What types of fruits are best?

There is hardly any information available online for people who exercise or train for sports and who want to eat raw foods. Thank you for all of your advice!! I'm currently reading The Raw Secrets, and I feel very lucky to have that information about raw food.

A: What an athlete needs more of is calories coming from carbohydrates. Increasing your intake of greens will not work for you — as they do not contain enough calories (energy). What you need more of right now is fruit. Of course, getting enough vegetable matter is important, overall, but in your case you are apparently under-consuming carbohydrates — which leads to hunger and cravings.

Eating 3000 Calories from Fruit

Q: *Hello. My language is not very good because I am from Poland, but, yes, I read all that did you sent to me. I know that you are correct about fruits and vegetables. For 6 years, I was vegan, and now I am full raw. I have seen much improvement! I eat 2 meals per day, because I know that my stomach needs rest, like others parts of my body. I found only one difficult thing: How do I get 3000 or more calories from fruits only? I eat 7 to 10 bananas for breakfast plus more fruits and greens, and then I eat something similar 5 hours before I am going to go to sleep. I am very active. I am running cycling and climbing, and I do a lot more exercises, which is why I want to know. Which fruits have a lot of calories?*

A: To get 3000 calories a day, I would personally recommend to work towards eating a 1500 calorie lunch as your main meal. Then, breakfast only needs to be 500 calories, and dinner could be around 1000 calories. That may seem like a lot of fruit, at first, so you may want to start with 4 meals a day.

You can later reduce to two. The following are some high calorie fruits that you could eat: mangoes, bananas, honeydew melon, figs, or persimmons.

If you're only going to eat 2 meals a day, then you will need to increase the amount of fruit per meal. The easiest way to reduce the load on your stomach with such a large amount of calories would be to blend yourself a few, large, high-calorie smoothies.

Eating Fruit and Running

Q: *I took the giant step towards a raw lifestyle about a month ago, and, while I'm not 100% raw yet, I feel great. I feel leaner, cleaner, and, just overall, better. My big concern is can a raw food diet maintain the fuel/energy requirements of an athlete. I'm a runner. I run about 30 miles a week and compete in races monthly, during the race season (mostly 1/2 marathons). Because I haven't been able to figure out the best way to carb load on a raw diet, I still have my bowl of pasta the night before. I'm afraid not to. Have you already addressed this in a previous article or series? If not, I think this would be a great topic for a future one! Thank you for making the raw foods way of life look so easy and delicious! The switch can be intimidating when you don't know what you are doing, and you make it look so simple.*

A: As an amateur runner myself, let me give you some tips. I don't run as much as you do, but I have done as much as 20 miles a week.

On a low-fat, high fruit diet, you're going to have much better results with your training. First of all, you don't need to "carb load", because fruits, unlike cooked complex carbohydrates, are easily digested and provide quick energy.

The problem with most runners is that they don't eat enough simple carbohydrates, which is what the body really needs when you're running.

The most important thing is to get enough calories and carbs overall. As a runner, you'll probably need to eat at least 3000 calories a day. That's about 30 bananas, or less, if you add in some vegetables and other varieties of fruit.

When I run longer than 90 minutes, I take some fruit with me, usually blended, seedless watermelon, or a smoothie made with water, bananas and celery, and drink that every 15 minutes.

You don't need to "carb load" when you're eating enough carbs (and most runners aren't, unfortunately).

For the best information, I recommend the book Nutrition and Athletic Performance, by Doug Graham. It will answer all of your questions and more.

How to Get More Calories

Q: *Help! I'm shrinking! I need serious support in eating more raw calories. I've been raw for almost three years now, and I have noticed weight loss to the point where I have no body fat. Are there specific recipes that are high in calories? I started having two big banana smoothies each day, but, in between, I'm not sure how to keep up. I have a very hectic life, working on film sets most of the time and non-stop lectures in grad school. Do you have any suggestions on how to boost calories? Specifically, what raw foods help to put on weight? Thanks so much. I love your cleanse and all the wonderful advice that you give. You've been my only support system in the transition to raw.*

A: I seriously doubt that you have "no" body fat. For a woman, a healthy body fat is between 11% and 20% or so and athletic males 3% to 9%, up to 12%. You should get that tested before making any assumptions. At your age, you probably have pretty high caloric requirements.

What you need is more fruit. Bananas are great, but there are many other high-calorie fruits, including:

• Mangoes

• Melons

• Durian (if available)

• Oranges (sweet varieties)

• Dates

• Figs

• Persimmons

• White nectarines or peaches

• As well as many tropical fruits: jackfruit, mamey, sapote, etc.

I have no idea what your "big" banana smoothie is. But I think my own diet should give you an example of what it takes to eat enough calories. I eat between 3000 and 3500 calories at the moment. And, likely, this is going to increase as I am training.

Breakfast:

Smoothie made with 4 cups of freshly squeezed orange juice, blended with 2 cups of mango flesh

Lunch:

7 extra-extra large bananas, blended with 2 cups of frozen wild blueberries

Dinner:

5 Haitian mangoes, pause of 30 minutes, then two huge blended salads consisting of:

• 3 large tomatoes

• 2 mangoes

• 6 cups of spinach

• 10 stalks of celery

• Juice of 1 lime squeezed on top

I have that blended salad in two sittings (two blendings)

I also have about 1 third of an avocado somewhere in there.

Total calories: over 3000, with about 6% coming from fat. Not that I worry about it, but the nutrients obtained is pretty much off the chart (including over 700mg of calcium), which is at least double the value for most requirements.

That was an extra-blended day! Normally, I don't have that much blended foods, but that really depends on what I feel like.

As you can see, to get enough calories, you have to eat A LOT. Personally, this kind of amount seems pretty normal to me. In fact, it's very satisfying and surprisingly easy to digest.

If you don't NEED to eat that much food, don't panic! Not everybody needs 3000 calories per day. The amounts will be dependent on your needs.

I also have to remind you that, although you need to eat enough calories to maintain your health, energy levels, and weight; in order to gain weight, you need to workout with weights 2-3 times a week. That's why you really need to figure out your true body fat soon. Go to a gym, and they will be able to tell you. Another possibility is to look online for a body fat measurement calculator and use a tape measure.

If it's not under 11% (for a woman) or 5% (for a man), then your body fat is NOT too low. What you need is more muscle!

You may find it easier to bring large quantities of cut up fruit or smoothies with you if you're always on the go. It's much faster to consume if it's already prepared for you.

How to Gain Weight

Q: *I am a Health Minister with Hallelujah Acres, which is an organization that I think you might be familiar with. They advocate eating some cooked food. I'm wondering if you have information on GAINING weight on a raw food diet. This is not for me. I try to eat all raw, but I have contact with an individual who is underweight and seems to think cooked food will address the problem. Do you have any suggestions?*

A: That's a very good question, but I think you're missing the point. First, you have to determine what is being "underweight"? Does that mean not having enough fat on you or not having enough muscle? Usually what happens is people lose a lot of body fat and then realize how under-muscled they are! In general, "underweight" people do not consume enough calories, especially on a raw food diet. In order to build muscle, you have to engage in weight training and lift heavy weights. You also have to make sure you're consuming enough calories for your muscles to grow. Eating more cooked food will not solve the problem. If the problem is an inadequate diet (not enough calories), you have to learn how to consume enough. A minimum for training individuals would be around 2000 calories for women and 2500 calories for men, per day. I suggest, in that case, that they:

• Track down calories consumed every day

• Incorporate strength training

• Make sure the diet is still low in fat and healthy

Afraid of Losing Weight On 100% Raw

Q: *I have read a lot about raw food eating, and I want to start it. However, I am afraid to lose weight, which happens every time that I eat less bread, grains, etc. Do you know of a person who had this problem, started eating 100% raw, and did not lose weight?*

A: I can only give you a generic response, keeping in mind that each situation is unique and must be dealt with on a case-to-case basis. It is easier to gain weight on bread, grains, and other cooked carbohydrates, because they are more concentrated in calories. For example, a few slices of bread will give you 500 calories, which would take 5 bananas or 10 peaches with raw foods. So the total volume that must be consumed, each day, on a raw food diet is much greater than on a standard cooked diet. The problem is that when people first go on a raw food diet, they start eating large quantities of fat (nuts, seeds, avocados, oil, etc.) to compensate. This leads to several health problems, and, possibly, for some people, the inability to gain weight, due to impaired digestion. I've known several people who couldn't gain sufficient weight on a typical high-fat, raw diet until they switched to a high-fruit, low-fat, raw diet. I, personally, have found that it is really easy to maintain my weight by eating only fruits and vegetables. At 5'10", I weigh about 158 pounds with a body fat level of about 12%. What I suggest that you to do is to figure out how many calories you actually need to maintain your weight. You do this using a simple calculation. - You take your ideal weight (the weight you'd like to achieve) and multiply by 10. - That will give you your "basic caloric requirements." - Then you add the calories you need for daily activities and for fitness activities. Take me for example:

- If my ideal weight is 145 pounds, then 1450 calories is the amount I need just to maintain my weight doing nothing.

- Then I need to add 300-400 calories for my daily activities, such as walking around the office, lifting up a few boxes of stuff, and so on. If someone is a postal office worker, or something like that, then you'll need to add a lot more for "daily activities." But I work most of the time on the computer.

- And then you add calories spent in fitness activities. For me, that's 500 to 1000 calories, depending on the day. So my total caloric intake should be about 2300 to 2800. Of course, all of this is very generic and depends on other factors, such as your total muscle mass, your age, etc., but this gives you an idea. Then you need to figure out how much food it actually takes to meet your caloric needs without getting more than 10-15% of your total caloric rom fat. To give you an idea, a banana generally yields 100 calories, and, ...-y big, it can yield up to 140 calories. So we're talking about a lot of fruit. For me, that means a breakfast of fruit, a lunch of fruit, and a dinner of fruit, followed by a giant salad or other vegetables. For a less active person, you could skip the fruit before the evening meal.

Salt and Sports

Q: *Thank you for your inspiring newsletters. I have a question about salt: For very active people is it important to replenish the body with salt after partaking in sports? I have low blood pressure, and I have noticed that I crave salt and get dizzy when I don't eat enough. But, lately, I've been adding more and more sea salt to my foods. How much salt is healthy?*

A: About salt: it's important to get enough sodium in the diet, but it's not necessary or recommendable to use table salt, sea salt, or Celtic salt. Active people need between 500 and 1000mg of sodium per day.

Greens contain the necessary sodium that we need. 1 stalk of celery contains about 50mg of sodium. A bunch of spinach contains almost 300mg. So it's not hard to get enough sodium; the key is to eat enough greens, probably about 1 pound or more a day, on average.

I suggest increasing the amount of greens, making green smoothies and blending celery with your fruit smoothies, instead of using sea salt or Himalayan salt. Please be aware that it's easy to take in too much sodium when using salt.

More than 1000 to 1500mg of sodium per day is unhealthy. Just a teaspoon of Celtic salt contains over 1500mg of sodium. You can already get at least 500mg from fruits and vegetables alone.

You also need to realize that the body uses the skin and elimination systems to get rid of excesses. People who eat spices like curry, garlic, or onions will also sweat some of it out through their skin.

Does this mean that they need to eat more of it because their body is getting rid of it? No. Most athletes that sweat out a lot of salt are ingesting a lot of salt in their diet, and the body is trying to get rid of it.

Still, all of these sports drinks include table salt and sugar, as if salt is just as important for muscle performance as glucose.

Chapter 7:
Families on a Raw Diet

Following the raw food diet on your own is one thing, but it becomes trickier when you have to view it in the context of your family and your entire social network.

Many people follow this raw-food lifestyle and wonder if this type of nutritional approach is correct during pregnancy or if they can feed their children raw foods only.

Because of important differences in humans, between our period growing up and our years as an adult, it's important to remember that the low-fat, raw food concept applies to fully-grown adults.

Because humans are designed to be breast-fed for a long period of time and human milk contains a fair quantity of fat (along with sugar, but surprisingly, very little protein), the suggestion of eating a maximum of 10% of total calories from fat does not apply to babies and children.

The most important thing for children is getting enough calories. A good variety of food is important (not just one category, like fruit or vegetables, but fatty foods such as nuts and needs should also be included).

Vitamin B12 is important, and a supplement should be included for pregnant and breast-feeding women as well as children.

I have not written the book on raw-food nutrition for children, but, in this chapter, I will attempt to answer some common questions on the subject, as well as address the social aspects of the raw-food lifestyle.

Babies on a Raw Diet

Q: *How does eating raw work for newly born babies, unfortunately, not on breast milk and beyond, such as a 1 and a half year old? Is there a healthy substitute for cow's milk other than soy? Are all raw foods okay for them? Are some better than others, and are some to be avoided?*

A: There are different opinions. Obviously, babies thrive on breast milk from healthy mothers, and there is no substitute that can be as healthy. If for any reason, the mother can't nurse, then I think the baby should have animal milk, ideally raw goat milk. If the option of a wet nurse is available, it would be a much better option.

Nut milks can be used as a healthful addition to the diet of babies, but not as the sole milk consumed.

Soft fruits can be introduced when the baby desires them. Although, at first, it will be just to satisfy curiosity.

At about 6 months of age, they can have fruit in addition to breast milk. Older than 6 months, blended fruits, green smoothies, and plain blended salads can also be introduced, and breast milk should still be the staple.

Other high-fat foods, such as coconuts, avocados, etc., can be introduced progressively.

Nuts can be introduced after 1 year, and they should be ground down or turned into milks Whole nuts and seeds should be avoided.

Foods to avoid would be salt, spices, garlic, sprouted beans, and raw starchy vegetables. Basically, most things that are not good for adults!

It should be noted that babies and young children need to eat more fat than adults (by percentage of total calories) to develop properly.

Breast-feeding on Raw

Q: I am currently breast-feeding a 4 month old baby, who receives no nutrition outside of my milk. I feel going raw would help many issues I am suffering. However, I am concerned that going raw would put me into detox and all the junk that I expel would go right into my baby's milk.

Do you have any advice on how slow I should transition or if I should forego trying to eat raw while nursing? It's been preached I need lots of whole grains when nursing and pregnant. Is that true?

A: I don't think that getting healthy is going to be harmful for yourself or your baby. What's the other option? Leaving all those toxins inside of your system?

I think that your body, in its infinite wisdom, will know what to do. I would not fear that toxins would go into your milk, and there is no evidence to show that this would happen, unless you're consuming toxins (like heavy metals) directly.

My suggestion is to get healthier now and not wait until later. Make sure that you are consuming at least 1 pound of greens a day, a lot of it in the form of blended greens, for optimal nutrition intake. Also of prime importance is making sure that you are consuming enough calories to produce quality milk. This means consuming enough fresh fruits, to get sufficient calories, and a limited amount of fat in the form of avocados, nuts, and seeds.

Grains are absolutely not necessary as long as you get enough calories from raw foods. Consuming a lot of grains is actually acid forming to your body, and all processed grains are fortified with artificial vitamins that aren't going to provide you with the proper nutrition that you can get from fruits and vegetables.

Protein Content of Breast Milk

Q: I'm a researcher by training. So when you said that human breast milk contains only 6% protein, I had to investigate this claim. If you check the American Pediatric Association website, you will find that it contains between 60% to 80% protein. I'm curious from what source(s) did you learn that human breast milk contains 6% protein? I've heard from Loren Lockman, who owns Tanglewood Wellness Center in Panama, claiming that human breast milk contains .025% protein. With due respect, I think your credibility would be enhanced if you would cite the sources of your findings.

A: Thanks for writing. You will see that I did not get my facts wrong! The only proper way to look at the percentage of protein in foods is to look at the percentage of total calories. The website you mention probably listed the percentage of protein by dry weight, which is completely misleading. If you enter "human milk" in any food database you will see that the percentage of protein per calories is only 6%. It would be impossible that this percentage could be 60%, as even cow's milk is only 26% of protein of total calories (and we all know it contains more protein than human milk, which is sweeter). Here's the information from fitday:

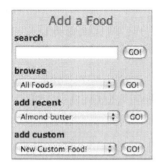

	grams	cals	%total
Total:		171	
Fat:	11	97	55%
Sat:	5	44	25%
Poly:	1	11	6%
Mono:	4	37	21%
Carbs:	17	68	39%
Fiber:	0	0	0%
Protein:	3	10	6%
Alcohol:	0	0	0%

Add a Food

search [ ] (GO!)

browse [All Foods] (GO!)

add recent [Almond butter] (GO!)

add custom [New Custom Food!] (GO!)

Calories Eaten Today

☐ Fat ☐ Carbs ☐ Protein ■ Alcohol

Today's Foods

Food Name	Servings	Serving Size	Cals	Fat	Carb	Prot
☐ Milk, human	1	cup	171	11	17	3
		Totals	171	11	17	3

(Save Changes) (Remove Checked)

Toxins in Breast Milk

Q: *I have been on your email list for a several months, and I have been watching all the notices about cleanses. I don't think that I can join, because I'm breast-feeding. I read that you don't want to detox while breast-feeding, because the toxins will come out in the breast milk and be bad for the baby. I have never seen you address this question. What is your take on it?*

Also, what do you suggest breast-feeding women do instead if they can't fast or detox? Because, you know, many women breast-feed almost constantly for 2, 4, 6 or more years in a row, depending on the number and spacing of their children.

A: First of all, the "cleanses" that I recommend are just really clean, good diets that you could follow for a very long time without problems. I'm not talking about taking any harmful products that would supposedly "cleanse" your body.

Let's look at it from a different point of view: Would it be harmful to not stop smoking before pregnancy, because you'd be afraid that the "detox" of the cigarettes would harm the baby?

Or would it be okay to continue drinking coffee or alcohol during pregnancy because going cold turkey would be too "dangerous" for the baby?

The answer of course is no. That's complete nonsense. It's always more harmful to continue a harmful habit during pregnancy than to discontinue it. The whole issue around detox has been completely exaggerated with no proof behind it whatsoever

I do not think that pregnant women or breast-feeding women should fast, but I also don't think that, if they did, it would pose health hazards to the baby.

Any weight loss at all will result in the breakdown of (according to you) fat-soluble toxins. That's what everybody says: Don't lose weight at all when you're breast-feeding, or fast at all, because it will release too many toxins into the bloodstream. But there is absolutely no evidence to support this.

From BabyCenter: "One study looked at women who had average exposure to environmental contaminants and an average loss of 4.1kg, between 4 and 20 weeks after the birth of their baby. The research found no link between a change in the women's body weight and contaminant concentration in their breast milk."

What is to be avoided is calorie-restricted diets or prolonged fasting. But moderate weight loss is healthy.

In fact, it's much better to CLEAN your diet and avoid toxins coming from the outside than to worry about stored toxins in your body that might be released if you lose body fat as you eat healthier or fast.

Recommended Reading for Raw-Vegan Pregnancy

Q: *Is there any book that can you recommend to me that you have written or any other article that I should read about raw-vegan pregnancy? Please let me know. Thank you.*

A: I have not written an article on the subject, because I simply do not have any type of experience on this. I did not think of covering this before, because I do not have children of my own. And I don't like to talk about things that I don't have any experience with.

But here are a few pointers that will certainly point you in the right direction:

1) The main thing during pregnancy and breast feeding is to get enough calories. Most raw-foodists are not consuming enough food. Under-eating is okay, for a while, if you need to release some weight. However, when you have a human being growing inside of you, you need to get enough nutrition. So I really recommend counting calories and making sure that you are getting enough foods.

2) Just be certain to get enough minerals from greens, I would also recommend either a few green smoothies a day, a big blended salad, or about 16 ounces of vegetable juice (mostly greens like celery, spinach, kale, and with a bit of carrot and lime for flavor, if you like). Salads are great, but most people don't chew well enough to assimilate all the nutrients.

3) Protein and fat is not more of an issue during pregnancy or breast-feeding than any other time. Again, what's important is to get enough calories from healthy sources. By doing so, you will have a sufficient balance of protein, fats, and carbohydrates.

4) Vegan doctors worldwide also recommend a Vitamin B12 supplement just in case.

5) Other factors of healthy living are just as important: sunshine, proper (safe) exercise, and enough sleep (crucial).

As for raising kids, there is more to say because nutritional requirements are a bit different for them, just in terms of the ratio of fat to carbs. But that is another topic.

Dealing with Hostile Friends and Family

Q: *Do you find yourself having to defend your rejection of drinking putrid tap water, or not wanting to eat a family dinner of dead pig and salt juice without getting abuse and offense? I'd love you to post some great comebacks for people's misinformed comments/insults, especially in regards to the good old staples of milk and cheese and the delightful, chemical-laden meat products.*

A: I don't mind people's opinions too much. With time and a little psychology, differences are better accepted. I don't think there are any good lines to throw at people when they challenge your beliefs. It will only make the situation worse. I find that the best approach is to instead agree with them, change the subject, or refer to the opinion of your doctor. I find it pointless to start a discussion, in most cases. Instead, be polite, smile, use psychology, and do not challenge.

Here are some examples:

"BUT WHERE DO YOU GET YOUR PROTEIN?!"

Wrong Answers: (Note: don't use these unless you insist on ruining the party and making a fool of yourself)

1) Where does the gorilla get its protein? Where does the cow get its protein? You know, this whole theory is wrong, you've been brainwashed, man!

2) I get my protein from fruit!

Better Answers: (Note: Do not challenge, just make friends. People who are interested will come to you.)

1) Actually, I don't really know. My doctor (or nutritionist) takes care of that.

2) Well, I find nutrition to be a very boring subject. By the way, did you see the new Tom Hanks movie?

3) I don't know. I never really thought about that. But, you know, I feel good; and that's the most important thing, don't you think?

"YOU KNOW, IF YOU DON'T DRINK MILK, YOU'LL GET OSTEOPOROSIS!"

Wrong Answers: (Note: do not use unless you're absolutely committed to making enemies.)

1) You know, we don't need to drink milk to get strong bones! It's all false propaganda by the milk industry!

2) Did you know that the 3 countries that have the highest rates of osteoporosis are also the biggest consumers of dairy products? What do you say to that!?

Better Answers: (Note: agree with something instead. You know that they're not ready to hear the truth anyway!):

1) Oh, well, I better check that out. Thanks for the advice.

2) You know, I used to think exactly that! By the way, did you see the new Tom Hanks movie?

"I READ IN THE NEWSPAPER THAT VEGETARIAN DIETS ARE DANGEROUS!"

Wrong Answer:

1) It's all a bunch of lies paid by the meat industry!

Better Answers:

1) Oh, really? I better check that out. Thanks. Would you pass me that bowl of guacamole?

2) Oh, really? Oh well, my doctor isn't too worried about that. He thinks it's helping me, so I trust him.

Remember, people think the opinion of a doctor is the Word of God, unless it's a vegan doctor of course.

That should give you some ideas for now. If you get trouble from your family and friends regarding your diet/lifestyle, send me the questions you get asked, and I'll come up with some answers for you in a future issue!

Raw Food for Pets

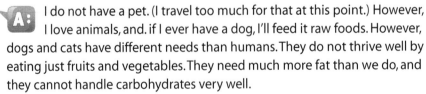

Q: *Do you have a dog or cat? If you do, I'm curious about what you feed them.*

A: I do not have a pet. (I travel too much for that at this point.) However, I love animals, and. if I ever have a dog, I'll feed it raw foods. However, dogs and cats have different needs than humans. They do not thrive well by eating just fruits and vegetables. They need much more fat than we do, and they cannot handle carbohydrates very well.

Cats should also be fed primarily meat, organs, bone marrow, etc. Their digestive tract is not designed for fruits and vegetables as they are natural carnivores.

There's a book on the subject that you can read. It's called Raw Dog Food. There are also several websites on the BARF diet for cats and dogs (BARF stands for Biologically Appropriate Raw Food). Just do a Google search for "Barf Diet" or "Raw Pet Food", and you'll find tons of information. Here's the website from the instigator of this method: www.drianbillinghurst.com

Traveling in the Raw! Family-Friendly, Raw Destinations

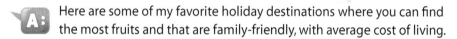

You have clearly had a lot of experience traveling and raw-foodism, could you possibly tell me where the best holiday destinations with the most fruit are that are also family friendly? (I am from New Zealand. So even seemingly "obvious" destinations (i.e. California??) would be very helpful!) Thank you so much! P.S. Thank you for all your info/books! Without them, I would still be eating a not-quite-so-SAD diet but not 100% raw!

Here are some of my favorite holiday destinations where you can find the most fruits and that are family-friendly, with average cost of living.

California: Great for the health food and raw scene. A car rental is usually a must to get around because of the large distances. There are lots of raw restaurants and the best, well-stocked, health food stores. Hotel room prices start at $100-130 for a decent room. Food costs are average for first world countries. A must visit if you're into raw-foods!

Hawaii: Great place to visit and easy to get around. There are some raw restaurants and good fruits at the farmer's markets and some good health food stores! Hotel room prices for a decent room are above $150. Food costs are higher than mainland USA.

Thailand: The ultimate place for fruit. It is very safe and children-friendly. Cheap accommodations and good rooms for families can be found at around $50, with other, more comfortable, higher-end options at prices far below North American (ultra-cheap, but clean rooms are also available in the $10-20 range). Food costs are very low, too.

Bali: My favorite island and still magical in spite of the tourism. It is super children-friendly. Lodging and food prices are only slightly above Thailand, but very affordable.

Costa Rica: Where I choose to live most of the year. It is great for families and nature lovers. There are lots of Bed and Breakfast types of rooms (where a fruit breakfast can usually be served). There are lots of fruit if you can drive to the farmer's market. It's a good idea to rent a car, or at least a driver, to see more of the country and be able to get fruit. I love the Southern Area (San Isidro + Dominical, Uvita, Quepos/Manuel Antonio). Families can rent a room for around $75-100, or less in most areas, but less expensive options are also available.

How to Eat Raw Traveling

Q: *We are planning a trip to Oaxaca, Mexico, this summer. Since I have been raw for over 3 years, I have yet to travel out of the country. So I am wondering if there are any concerns with eating raw in Mexico. I have always heard that you should only drink bottled water in foreign countries, but what, if any, precautions should I take in selecting my fruits and vegetables? Since you have done a lot of traveling, any information will be appreciated.*

A: What tends to happen is that people get sick from eating restaurant foods, or spiced local foods, when they travel. I have traveled in many tropical countries, and I have always stayed healthy when eating local fruits and vegetables. The only times that I became sick was when I ate local cooked foods because of too much salt, too many spices, or possible contamination. So my recommendation is to eat fruits and vegetables. All fruits that you can peel are great. And in Mexico that won't be a problem. This includes mangoes, bananas, sapote, papayas, and all the others. As for vegetables, I don't see a problem with vegetables sold at the market. I've never had problems with that. The vegetables that can make you sick are those that are prepared in a restaurant. I also recommend drinking only bottled water as tap water isn't as clean there.

Chapter 8:
Other Diet Programs

It would be fair to say that with every possible kind of diet out there, each claiming to be the best, the field of nutrition is rather confusing.

We also know that there's a state of mass confusion in the raw-food, vegan movement, and I'm willing to bet on the fact that you're probably still wondering who's right and who's wrong.

Let's face it: it can get pretty confusing. There is so much contradicting information about health and nutrition out there, that it's sometimes hard to separate the wheat from the chaff.

Sometimes, we wonder: Is there really truth among all of that, or is it up to the individual to "find out what works for him/her"?

In this chapter, I answer more questions about various diets and other claims made by different authors.

100% Raw or Steamed Vegetables

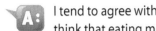 *I'm a believer in the benefits of raw. However, I came across this information by Dr. Joel Fuhrman, author of Eat to Live, a very well respected doctor who wrote this article on "The Cold Truth about Raw Foods". It makes a lot of sense to me: http://www.diseaseproof.com/archives/healthy-food-the-cold-truth-about-raw-food-diets.html*

What's your opinion on this? I think 100% raw is difficult to do, especially in a cold climate like Toronto. Thanks.

A: I tend to agree with the general position of Dr. Fuhrman. Although, I do think that eating more raw foods will give you better health results overall.

The question of "cooking" is actually quite secondary. The first question is: what are our natural foods?

The answer is simple: fruits and vegetables are our natural foods, best adapted to human physiology.

Then we also find that, in general, eating foods in their raw, natural state yield more benefits. There are some exceptions, as Dr. Fuhrman pointed out.

It then becomes a personal decision: do you eat 100% raw, or do you include steamed vegetables and other *relatively healthy* cooked foods into your diet as well? Personally, I still sometimes eat these items if ripe fruit isn't available. But the bulk of my diet is raw, and that's what I try to stick to.

What I find in general is that once people open the door to cooked foods, then the rules become quite loose. Eventually, they're back to eating pretty much anything. It's often much easier to just stick with raw foods.

Also, a lot of the issues around absorption of the nutrients in vegetables can be solved by including blended salads and green smoothies into your diet. In a future post, I will describe an easy way to add more easily digestible raw vegetables to your diet.

Bottom line is if you eat some steamed vegetables, it's not the end of the world; and they could have some nutritional benefits. But, overall, raw foods are superior.

Are Humans Supposed to Eat Meat?

 Just a sincere legitimate question: Are humans supposed to eat meat? I have been reading the material of a lot of respected sources, including Steve Pavlina and your own site, but there are also some respected sites that stipulate quite the contrary, that meat and fats are good for human health. One example of the type of people that thrive are the Eskimos that live healthy on almost fatty meat and cite that in the glacial Era there were little fruits.

I have found compelling, respected evidence with citations and references of *both* that humans are natural carnivorous and herbivorous.

Some sites/books even say that most of our calories should come precisely from fat.

There are also comments that the meat ingestion was responsible for the growth and evolution of the human brain.

Please help me with this issue, as the two theories are quite opposite and cite the other to be not only neutral but dangerous.

How can I know which is right?

You seem like an honest health seeker, and, in fact, I remember clearly being exactly where you are right now.

Let's take a look at the issue and see if you can understand my own point of view on this.

So the question is: are humans supposed to eat meat? And is our ideal diet high in fat or high in carbohydrates?

First, let's start with the Eskimos. Although prior to the arrival of western civilizations, they were living in pretty robust health, the Eskimos are not reputed to have a very high life expectancy.

The lowest figure that I have heard was 35 years. The highest was not much higher than our current life expectancy.

On the other hand, the three, longest-lived cultures in the world, known in the last 100 years have been:

The Vilcambaba in Ecuador, the Abkhasia in Russia, and the Hunzas in Pakistan.

All of these cultures, without exception, have lived on a low-fat diet with limited supply of meat and animal products.

As for the growth of the human brain, to me it's completely ludicrous that this came from eating meat. The researchers who came up with that are lost in their own wonderland of romantic thinking about the strong hunter-gatherers and cave-men, who dragged their female partners by the hair to their caves and from whom we supposedly evolved.

Just look at the model in nature.

The most intelligent of all apes are the ones that eat the most fruit. Bonobos are the most intelligent of all the great apes, and they're the ones eating the most fruit and the least animal products.

It seems to me that it is more obvious that fruit eating has a direct relationship with the intelligence in animal species, rather than meat eating.

After all, the carnivores are not necessarily the smartest creatures around, compared to the smart frugivores.

Think about it: An orangutan must have knowledge of over 150 species of fruit and plants to survive. It not only knows which fruits are in season, but can precisely time its eating patterns to specific trees in a rather large area where it lives. As one fruit tree goes out of season in one area, it knows that another variety somewhere else far away is about to go into season. And all that without calendars!

To me, being a frugivore in nature requires a lot more intelligence than hunting for meat. And that's why I think our brains evolved by eating large quantities of fruit and maybe root vegetables as they are high in calories, as that was an early "cooked food" staple in many tribes. But eating meat just isn't as prevalent as society is accustomed to today.

Also, humans will survive on ANYTHING!

And all of the primitive diets are healthier than the Standard American Diet for a very good reason. They avoid four of the main culprits that make our own diet so bad. These are:

• Bread and gluten containing products

• Refined dairy products

• Caffeine

• Processed foods, sugar, condiments, and preservatives

Just put anyone on any diet that eliminates these categories of foods, and they'll get better. There's no doubt about it. In my book *The Raw Secrets*, I describe in detail, the reasons why we are meant to eat a low-fat, high-fruit diet and how to best thrive on this diet.

Why not give it a try? Do you honestly believe that killing animals and eating their flesh is what humans are supposed to eat to best thrive on?

What about the fact that our entire system is NOTHING like that of a carnivore or an omnivore. Our entire system matches that of the frugivore, from our teeth to digestive tract.

I will agree with you that the traditional, vegan diet which contains a lot of bread, wheat products, refined foods, soy, and fat is not healthy.

This is not what I'm proposing here. I endorse a raw vegan diet, composed mainly of fruits, vegetables, nuts, and seeds.

If you need more scientific evidence on the animal products issue, read some well-researched books such as:

The China Study

Eat to Live

These are the two books that I recommend. They're not raw-food books, but they have some very important information on the subject of animal consumption.

Blood Type Diet and Superfoods

Q: *I'd just be curious to get your opinion on 2 matters. You've talked briefly about other diets, but I was wondering, what was your take on the blood type diet? Given that I'm O+, I'm naturally "supposed" to be a carnivore. So I was wondering, if by being vegan, I was going against my body's natural instincts. Is there any logical and reasonable rationale behind that diet?*

Secondly, I was just wondering what you thought of "superfoods", such as maca, chlorella, etc. Are they the real deal, or are they just false hype? Given that I put a ridiculous amount of stress on my body (amateur cycling training, working night shifts, etc.), I'm always on the lookout for new ways to take care of my body (the five Tibetan rites are working wonders). Thank you very much for your time, and keep up the good work.

1) The blood type diet issue has been discussed before in some articles that I have published. But here's my take on it: I have a lot of experience studying that diet. In fact, I was even in close contact with one of the foremost promoters of this diet, here in Canada.

I have read all of the books, and I have been to every website that promotes it. After reviewing all of that information, I came to the conclusion that the blood type diet is based on very weak evidence. There is no real scientific evidence to prove that certain blood types must eat meat while others should not.

It is true that our blood type is part of our genetic makeup and that there is some evidence to show that some blood types are more prone to certain diseases, but there is absolutely no evidence to show that certain blood types should eat totally different diets.

Consider this: different kinds of animals have different kinds of blood types, yet they all eat the same foods. Dogs have 4 different blood types, cats have 11 blood types, and cows about 800. However, you'll never see a cow eating like a cat!

The biggest differences in metabolism in humans are found between men and women, yet no one so far has come up with a "man's diet" and a "woman's diet", in which each gender should eat completely different foods!

There is as much evidence to prove the validity of the blood type diet as there is to prove the validity of astrological predictions. In fact, the idea that our blood type influences our personality is so popular that in Japan people ask, "What's your blood type?" like we ask, "What's your sign"?

2) For the most part, superfoods are 95% hype. I have found that most "superfoods" are in fact "super-stimulants" and not a real source of energy. If you place tremendous stress on your body in terms of increased physical activity and working at night, then you need more rest. But, unfortunately, there's no "superfood" that's going to compensate for the lack of sleep. And, of course, there's no money in saying that.

Blood Types and the Raw Food Diet

 Please comment if there are some blood types that aren't compatible with living foods. What is your blood type?

 There is absolutely no reason to believe that any restrictions must be placed on the foods that you eat based on your blood type. This entire theory is unfounded.

Many animal species have different blood types, yet they eat essentially the same foods. Cows have 800 different blood types, and yet they all thrive on the same diet!

The "blood type" diet is often a good excuse for people to explain their failures on the raw food diet, when it is easily explainable for other reasons.

Knowing my blood type won't add any weight to this discussion. I know successful raw-foodists of all blood types: A, B, AB and even the meat-eating "O".

Breatharianism

 What do you think about breatharianism? There is an interview with a person who claims to live on nothing but air and distilled water!

 Before I answer this reader's question about "breatharianism", I want to tell you a breatharian joke.

A group of people go to a "breatharian" restaurant.

The waiter comes and asks the first person, "What will you have sir?"

The first breatharian answers, "I'll get a cold breeze of arctic air."

Then the waiter asks the second person what she'd like.

She answers, "I'll take some warm, mint-perfumed, tropical air."

"All right, he answers, and what about you sir? "The waiter asks the last person in the group.

The last man replies, "Oh, nothing for me today. I'm fasting."

Ok, I admit. That was a really bad joke.

There are a lot of people claiming a lot of crazy things. Personally, my experience with these so-called breatharians has not proven to me that living on nothing but air and water is a possibility.

I believe it's possible for a person to get to a state where they actually need to consume very little food, but I don't believe that this is a healthy practice as a lifestyle, nor that it is possible to actually "live on air" indefinitely.

I met my first "breatharian" in California about 10 years ago, and the person in question is probably the most famous "breatharian" at the moment.

She seemed frail, and she was actually fighting a cold when I met her. She got paid pretty decent money (over $5000) to give a one-day talk on "living on light", with all expenses paid. She had just bought a new house, and she seemed to be doing well being a breatharian "guru".

I was pretty shocked when she said that this "lifestyle" was great for teenagers, because with all the money they saved by not eating, they could spend more money on clothes!

The whole thing seemed pretty ludicrous, especially when she revealed actually eating chocolate cookies, tea with soy milk, pasteurized orange juice, and other non-foods just for the "taste" and not for the nutrition.

My belief is that these "breatharians" simply get by with eating very little, but, eventually, all of them end up eating to sustain themselves.

This famous breatharian has actually accepted in 1999 to be challenged by Australia's 60 Minutes. She was willing to not eat and drink for one week to prove her methods.

After just a few days, she became severely dehydrated, listless, and gaunt, and lost a tremendous amount of weight. The "experiment" was aborted for health reasons.

The breatharian, of course, blamed it on "polluted air" that prevented her from getting the nutrients. What a joke!

I also met another famous breatharian, actually, probably the most famous of all, Wiley Brooks. He greeted me like this, "Hi, I'm Wiley Brooks, the breatharian."

From what I gathered from people who knew him personally, Wiley had no problem eating a hamburger once in a while, and he was actually caught, more than once, entering a fast food joint.

He claims that this food is simply to fulfill his need for "pleasure" and "taste", and it is not what keeps him alive.

To finish the topic, I know of several people who have died when trying to become breatharians. Closer to me, I have met several people who have gone to these extremes of "purity" in their diet, and one of them actually died.

In my opinion, breatharianism is a complete fraud and anyone promoting this idea should really look at the potential harm it's doing to its followers.

Frugal Eating

Q: *Your best-kept secret from last issue was very interesting. But I keep thinking that the greatest health secret is the one exposed by Cornaro: eat and drink as little as possible. Cornaro consumed one liter of liquid per day and one pound of food. He ate of everything (eggs, meat, etc.). But the principle of frugality seems to be very important to me, even of prime importance. What do you think?*

A: Regarding frugality, it mostly helps those who have an unhealthy diet. The consequences of the traditional diet lessen when one practices frugal eating. They can then live longer and in better health.

But someone eating mostly fruits and vegetables will need to eat much more to sustain an active lifestyle. Those foods are not concentrated, so we need to eat more to fulfill our needs.

If we try to restrict ourselves, we may well fall into worse mistakes. Not eating enough is a common mistake of people who attempt to follow a raw diet. It's important to eat enough for our energy needs. But with a Standard American Diet, I agree that frugal eating helps. Eating less of a toxic substance is healthier than eating more of it.

How Do You Know if The Raw Diet is the Right Diet?

Q: *How do you know if the raw diet is right, when it is a relatively new 'diet'? Have any large groups of people lived on a raw food diet in the last century and lived a healthier existence? Where's the proof? Is there any statistical evidence to support this diet?*

What about those people that live to be 90 and above on a cooked food diet?

What do you say to that? How old do you expect you will live for?"

A: You're bringing what I call a more "philosophical question", so I'll be as honest as possible with you.

There has been a lot of research to prove that the healthiest diet is a plant-based diet. You can refer to the extensive research quoted by Dr. Fuhrman, Dr. Klaper, Dr. Barnard, T. Colin Campbell, and many others. The best book to consider on the subject is called Eat to Live by Dr. Fuhrman. Another book to consider is the China Study by T. Colin Campbell.

There is not a lot of "statistical" data that a completely raw vegan diet is the best, because, as you aptly pointed out, there haven't been large groups of identifiable people following this diet. And no one is paying to fund these studies.

Just in the raw food movement alone, the differences of applications in the diet are completely different! For example, a fruit-based, raw food diet is completely different nutritionally than a fat-based (nuts and oil), raw food diet.

The truth is; we're pioneers. And true pioneers have arrows in their backs. There isn't a lot of support for this diet, because it flies in the face of the food pyramid and what's recommended by the FDA!

But you can consider the following:

1- A mostly raw or all raw diet with sufficient calories is the most nutrient dense diet on the planet.

2- Eating mostly or only raw foods makes sense on many levels. Even mainstream nutritionists tell us that fruits and vegetables are the healthiest foods.

3- Just notice how you feel. Don't you feel better on a low-fat, raw food diet compared to a mainstream diet?

4- Thousands of people are regaining their health and their lives with the raw food diet. Most people report extreme improvements in energy levels, mood, body fat levels, and health in general.

Yes, there are people who reach the age of 90 eating a mainstream diet. But you have to understand that diet isn't the only factor in longevity! Many factors are important, and include the following: genetic predispositions, stress, active lifestyle, not overeating, a simple lifestyle, and a general state of mind. When these people die, eating a mainstream diet, it is also because something is overloaded and fails, or their immune system is so poor that a mild cold or flu kills them.

If you think that you have a good chance of making it to 90 in good health on a Standard American Diet, consider this:

- Most people over the age of 40 take medications, and almost everybody over the age of 60 takes drugs and has some sort of degenerative disease.

- The cancer rates in this country are increasing every year, in spite of advances in medicine for the treatment.

- The new generation, which are children born from my generation, are sicker than any generation before. More children have or develop serious health problems in the first years of their lives than in my generation or the generation of my parents or grand-parents.

- Increased life-expectancy is a myth. My generation is sicker than my parent's generation and will likely live less long, and, for the children of my generation, it will be even worse.

I personally don't expect to live to be 100 or even 90. I'm not being pessimistic but realistic. I didn't inherit the strongest health and constitution, and I was raised on lots of junk food like most people.

But I'm 100% convinced that by taking care of my health, I will live longer and stay healthier than if I kept eating a Standard American Diet. Who knows what would have happened to me, even by now!

Don't be a fool to think that your friends are doing just fine on a Standard American Diet. Almost everyone who eats a standard diet is sicker than they'd like to admit.

Here's the honest truth: the raw food diet and lifestyle can be a very healthy lifestyle. It won't guarantee that you'll live to be 100. It won't solve all of your problems. It won't make you 100% healthy, and it won't be always easy.

But if you give it a try, stop spending your time in doubt and fear, and actually do it, I believe your own experience with it will be the best proof to you that it works.

No Fruit Diets and the Glycemic Index

Q: *I think you need to address the low-glycemic movement in the raw food world. Hippocrates and Tree of Life advocate little to no fruit to improve health. Why go with more fruits when these reputable health centers say no?*

A: I do not find the glycemic index to be a very useful chart overall. Essentially, to create this index they measured the "average" blood sugar response in "average" people, after eating different types of food.

The key word is "average".

The average person does not exercise, is overweight, and eats a high fat diet. So the results of the glycemic index tables will only reflect how the average person reacts to food, not necessarily how a healthy person reacts.

That being said, it's clear that some foods produce a higher glycemic response than others. This is where the glycemic index can be useful. For example, watermelon raises blood sugar much faster than apples. So it could be your food of choice when you are exercising or after coming back from the gym, when you need to raise your blood sugar, after depleting it through exercise.

Relatively speaking, the glycemic index of watermelon is still fairly low compared to most other foods, and almost all fruits are low to moderate on the index. If you're eating a low-fat raw food diet, you should have no problems with stable blood sugar, regardless of what fruit you are eating if it is not combined with fatty foods.

As for the centers you mention, I could go on and on about this and explain to you in detail why fruit is not the problem. Start by reading my "Shocking Report on the Fruit Controversy" at www.fredericpatenaude.com/fruitreport.pdf

I believe that the concept of eating little to no fruit to improve your health is an aberration. Literally, every single truly reputable health professional on the planet recommends fruits and vegetables for health. Also all primates are frugivores and consume massive quantities of fruits and greens, abstaining from all grains and cooked foods, and they have no blood sugar issues.

The following doctors and researchers also recommend a high-carbohydrate, low-fat diet, based upon thousands and thousands of scientific studies:

• Dr. T. Colin Campbell (China Study)

• Dr. Douglas Graham (80-10-10 Diet)

• Dr. Joel Fuhrman (Eat to Live, also a high-fruit diet)

• Dr. John McDougall (McDougall Program, only 7% fat)

• Dr. Dean Ornish (Ornish Program for heart disease)

• Dr. Neal Barnard (From Physician Committee of Responsible Medicine)

• Dr. Alan Goldhamer (The Pleasure Trap)

• And many others

I do not doubt that people who visit the "low-fruit" centers that you recommend experience health benefits. However, it is not necessarily because they are avoiding fruit. It is because of the other healthy changes that they make from their previous lifestyle.

They are eliminating meat, dairy, fast food, refined food, reducing sodium intake, and increasing their hydration. It's no doubt that they are experiencing health benefits when they remove the cause for so many adverse health conditions. You can do all of this yourself without the help of a health center by choosing to eat fresh fruits and vegetables instead of the "Standard American Diet".

As I have demonstrated elsewhere, a low-fruit, 100% raw diet is a very HIGH fat diet. There is no credible evidence or research that encourages such a high fat diet.

It is also not possible to design a no-fruit, low-fat, 100% raw food diet. You have to get calories from somewhere, vegetables and greens have negligible calories so you will either be eating a large amount of fruit or nuts, avocados and oils. Fats are denser and calories add up much quicker than the same volume of food in fruit. Fruit is mostly comprised of water for proper hydration; fats are not. What sounds healthier to you?

What about a Low Glycemic Diet?

Q: *And, last, but not least, when discussing the optimal diet, one of the criteria listed was that it be "low glycemic". Again, this gets back to the fruit issue, as many fruits are high glycemic. So, again, even though I love fruit, I'm beginning to wonder just how wise it is to consume it on a regular basis.*

A: Most fruits are not "high" on the glycemic index. Banana is 51 (low), Kiwi is 47 (low), Grapefruit is 25 (low), Mango is 41 (low), Oranges is 31 (low), Papaya is 56 (low). Only watermelon is listed as "high" on most charts (72).

According to Dr. Fuhrman, author of the excellent book Eat to Live, "Scientific evidence indicates that the glycemic index of a food is not a reliable predictor of the effect food has on blood glucose levels, cholesterol, and insulin levels."

You need to not be concerned about the glycemic index of a particular food if it is otherwise nutrient and fiber-rich. The presence of fiber in whole fruits is much more important in blood glucose control than the glycemic index.

Even high-glycemic carbohydrates, such as grains, (which I do not recommend anyway), will not cause blood sugar problems or diabetes if they are consumed whole and in the context of a low-fat diet.

Those high-glycemic foods are linked to glucose intolerance and insulin insensitivity, or insulin resistance (the inability for insulin to properly "carry" sugar to the cells) when consumed with excessive quantities of FAT.

Due to the consumption of high-fat foods, there's a lack of insulin receptors in the cell surface, and high levels of insulin are secreted.

When carbohydrates, including sweet fruits, are consumed without fat, and in the context of a low-fat diet, they cause a rather low insulin response.

When someone decides to follow a low-glycemic index diet, they may even be causing diabetes if they are eating more high-fat foods that cause the body to secrete more insulin because of insulin resistance.

The glycemic index is also very imprecise, because the effect of the same foods on different people can be so different that it would be wrong to consider the glycemic index charts accurate in the first place.

Fruits and vegetables are low to moderate; some being a bit high on the glycemic index. However, this doesn't even matter. Even high glycemic index foods, such as potatoes, have no incidence on diabetes and sugar-metabolic disorders in the context of a low-fat diet. Many cultures have a 0% incidence of diabetes, and their diet is composed of 80% high-glycemic foods, such as potatoes or rice.

People who write about diets and tell people NOT to eat certain fruits and vegetables because they are supposedly "high-glycemic," or because of some other issue, such as "hybridization" or "natural fructose", are scaring people away from natural foods and instead promote things like raw butter and grass-fed beef. It's sad.

Natural, whole foods are ALWAYS better than refined foods, and it doesn't matter where they fit on a glycemic chart that some scientists made up, using unhealthy people, eating a Standard American Diet as their point of reference. I, personally, do not rely on flawed charts and incorrect theories to feed myself, and I encourage you to do the same.

Traditional Diets and Longevity

Q: I like the no nonsense advice that you give, and much of it made real sense to me. I am currently not all raw and may never be, and here is why: Have you heard of the 25-year Okinawan study? These are the oldest centenarians on our planet. They eat cooked food, mostly grain, along with fermented vegetables, soy products, some fruit, very little dairy, and about 5 to 10% meat (mostly fish high in Omega 3 oils). So, I am wondering: why all raw? If there is evidence that traditional diets are healthy and healing, then why not follow them and make sure that you do get some raw food as well? Dr. Walford, MD, of the BioSphere 2 fame (a two year project in the Arizona desert), proved that a low-calorie, high nutrient diet is beneficial for reducing disease/illnesses and extending life. Again, why all raw if I don't live in a tropical zone? Why not follow a traditional diet that will keep me disease free and healthy?

 I do not recommend traditional diets, and here is why:

The most important thing is to eat primarily foods that are specific to humans. Those are fruits and vegetables. Traditional diets are high in grains, and those foods are not specific to humans. A high-grain diet will cause all sorts of problems. Please refer to my book for more information or check out Grain Damage by Dr. Doug Graham.

You cannot attribute the longevity of these people solely on diet. You can generally attribute it to:

1) Frugality - eating little food (which lessens the impact of non specific foods)

2) Stress free life

3) An active lifestyle

4) Good quality foods (No GMOs or pesticides, etc.)

5) Good genetics

If you follow a traditional diet yourself, you will not live as long as those people, because you are not under the same circumstances.

A traditional diet is better than the Standard American Diet, but it is not the best, nonetheless. If those people ate specific foods (fruits and vegetables), and less or no grains, dairy, etc., I am quite certain that they would live even longer.

When researchers find a group of centenarians, the first thing that they do is they look at their diet and attribute their longevity to something that they eat. Usually, the centenarians themselves will attribute their longevity to something they eat. "I'm healthy because I eat beef broth." Or, "I'm healthy because I eat bone marrow." They'll claim that centenarians in Eastern Europe live longer because they eat kefir. But centenarians in other parts of the world do not eat kefir, and they live just as long. Could it be that all of those foods have nothing to do with their longevity?

Could it be that they live longer not because of the kefir, but in spite of it? I dare to say so.

A low-calorie diet will extend life for the good reason that it imposes frugality on its dieters. That limits, dramatically, the impact that non-specific foods (grains, etc.) will have on the body. But, when eating mostly fruits and vegetables, you can and should eat more calories.

As for raw versus cooked, it is not necessary to eat all raw if the only cooked foods you eat are steamed vegetables, for example. But, if you eat a mostly cooked diet of grains, vegetables, soy, dairy, and some meat, like the Okinawans, your health won't be as good as if you eat a fruits and vegetables based diet.

You can test it for yourself and see.

Again, what explains the longevity of those people are the factors that I've mentioned, but it's also the fact that their diet is better than most people, just not as optimal as it could be.

PS: If you were to have an orangutan as a pet, what would you feed it? Would you feed it grains and dairy, because you don't live in a tropical environment? No, you'd feed it its natural diet: fruits and vegetables. It's the same for us. It doesn't matter that we live in the north. Our physiology is the same, and it thrives best on a fruit and vegetable based diet.

Is Under-eating Healthy?

What do you think of "under-eating"?

Dr. Gabriel Cousens writes, "The most important single rule in nutrition is to under-eat!" He continues, "This rule takes precedence over all other dietary advice… In experiments with animals, the under-eaters in general, were more youthful, vigorous, and energetic, when compared to normals, and showed minimal to no chronic degenerative diseases."

First of all, let's define OVEReating. I think pretty much everyone agrees that overeating is eating beyond one's caloric needs. So using the same definition, UNDER-eating just means eating below one's caloric needs.

Is that good? How could eating less food than what the body needs be healthy?

What these authors mean when they talk about "under-eating" as being a healthy practice, they simply refer to eating less concentrated and refined food.

It doesn't mean eating less fruits and vegetables or restricting oneself on the quantity of fruits and vegetables eaten.

Most of the experiments that concluded that under-eating increases lifespan were done on laboratory animals eating concentrated refined foods. The wrong conclusion of these studies is that eating less of EVERYTHING is somehow good for health.

If you're a lab mouse and you're being fed the kind of diet that lab mice get, then you're probably going to live longer on half of the stuff!

If you're a human on the Standard American Diet, then you're also probably going to live a lot longer if you just cut the quantities of food in half.

However, if most of what you eat is fruits and vegetables, then you'll need to physically eat MORE. Why? That's because fruits and vegetables are not very concentrated in calories, but they are concentrated in nutrients. So, to get enough energy, you eat more food, but, at the same time, you get more nutrients.

This concept is called "nutrient density". It just means that it's healthier to eat foods that give you more nutrients per calorie "dollar". So 1000 calories of fruits and vegetables are going to give you a lot more nutrients than 1000 calories of bread and meat.

With whole fruits and vegetables, it would be very hard to overeat, since those foods are water-rich and nutrient-dense. However, it's quite common to under-eat. Thus, you can be hungry all the time, lose too much weight, and so on. This kind of under-eating is certainly not a good thing when trying to maintain a healthy, active lifestyle.

But, a standard diet is so toxic and concentrated that just by reducing the amount of food that you eat, you are certain to improve your health.

Chapter 9:
Specific Raw Foods Revealed

I get a lot of questions about specific foods on the raw food diet. So, in this chapter, I will answer some of the many questions that I've received about various raw foods.

One point that I want to make clear is that I don't subscribe to the idea that raw foods have specific "healing powers".

The body always does the healing, and what we can best do is assist it by giving it proper nutrition and avoiding the causes of disease.

Not only do raw foods NOT have any special powers, but also just eating more raw foods is not enough to make you healthy.

The raw food diet is very effective, not because of the foods that you eat, but because of the foods that you DON'T eat.

So just adding some fresh juices or fruit to a diet, which contains plenty of disease-forming foods (such as animal products and refined foods), will do very little to improve your health.

The trick is to eliminate the junk AND eat more raw foods.

Açaí

Q: *Have you ever tried açaí berry? What are your thoughts on purchasing it as a juice/concentrate? Thanks.*

A: I have eaten Açaí when I visited Brazil in 2004. For those who don't know, Açaí (pronounced AH-SAW-EE) is a slightly fatty, antioxidant-rich fruit that grows in Brazil. The Brazilians buy it frozen in big blocks. They make a national dish by blending it with either honey or guarana syrup, and they serve it with granola. Prepared that way, it is delicious. However, its recent use as "miracle food" is deplorable. People buy it at a 10 or 20 times markup.

Even though Açaí is a decent food, it's not necessary to eat it to stay in great health. There are other great, antioxidant-rich foods that are available, such as blueberries or pomegranates, which you can buy fresh and in season. You don't need to pay an outrageous price for this exotic juice.

If Açaí were available frozen at a reasonable price, then I would suggest making some sorbets with it, similar to what Brazilians make.

Is Algae Vegan?

Q: *Please let me know if I, as a raw vegan, can eat spirulina and seaweeds (wakame, arame, nori, dulse etc.), because I am not sure if they are plants or animals and if you recommend them for good health.*

A: Seaweed (including wakame, dulse, and nori) is a plant. Blue-green algae is classified by biologists in the group of "prokaryotae" -- apart from other groups: animalia (animals), fungi, plantae (plants) and protista (protists) -- although some also consider it to be part of either the protist or plant kingdom. So blue-green algae is not an animal, but it's not quite a plant either.

Some people like algae, but I find it to be a stimulating food and not a real source of nutrients. Instead of consuming algae, I encourage people to consume green, leafy vegetables, which are our true source of minerals.

As for seaweed, I do not recommend it on a daily basis, although I do consume some only occasionally (nori, dulse, or kelp). The problem with seaweed is that it contains a lot of excess salt, and, as with anything that comes from the sea, it is likely to contain some contamination from heavy metals, like mercury, which could outweigh any "benefits" from consuming it as a nutrient source.

Bean Sprouts

Q: *I would like to add sprouts to my diet for some variety. However, I'm having trouble finding food-combining advice for sprouts. What category are fresh bean (lentil, pea, chickpea, mung bean, adzuki bean) sprouts in? Are they fatty? Starchy? Simple sugary? Can they be combined with soaked nuts or other fats? I know that the stage of sprouting that they're in is relevant; I eat them when they have small, non-leafy tails of a few millimeters.*

Also, at what frequency do you recommend eating them?

A: First, I would like to say that I generally do not recommend the consumption of bean sprouts, except very rarely and in small quantities. Bean sprouts still contain a large amount of raw starch which is very difficult to digest. They also contain a number of enzyme inhibitors, which makes them very hard to digest as well as slightly toxic.

The kinds of sprouts that I recommend are the green sprouts, which are seeds that have fully sprouted into a small plant. Those include: sunflower greens, alfalfa, pea shoots, clover, fenugreek (in small quantities), and other sprouts that have a green leaf. Those sprouts can be considered vegetables and can be combined as vegetables. You can eat them as often as you desire.

Blended Salads

Q: *In your last newsletter issue, you say that blended salads are not for raw food beginners. Why not? I don't see the point of blending salads. Humans need to use their teeth!*

A: I said that blended salads are not for "beginners" simply because they won't be visually appealing to most people who are just getting started!

You are perfectly right. Humans need to use their teeth. However, let me point out several challenges here:

1- We have poor dental health. Name a person that you know who never had a cavity in their life? With all their wisdom teeth? With a perfect jaw structure from birth? I've rarely met such people.

The reality is that we often have compromised teeth. Remember that when you get dental work done, your teeth are never quite the same after. If you had your wisdom teeth pulled out, you are missing a major chewing area.

If your teeth are not completely in alignment (like in most people), you are never going to be able to chew completely well, like you would if your teeth and dental health had been perfect.

Remember, raw vegetables have to be completely chewed and turned into a liquid in order to be digested.

2- Monkeys spend 6 hours a day chewing. If you were to sit down and eat a salad big enough to really feed you and then try to chew it very, very well, you'd spend a long time chewing! Most people are not ready to do that, and, when they are, they might have dental issues as well.

So my point is not that you should stop chewing, but you need to understand that we're in a compromised situation here. If we want to get optimal nutrition from raw foods, we need to include blended foods in our diet, such as green smoothies or blended salads.

That doesn't mean you that can't have a nice salad, too, or eat fruit.

All the things that I've talked about - green smoothies, blended salads - are not meant to "replace" chewing but, simply, to be something that you might consider adding to your diet.

Dulse

Q: *I have some colitis and have had some bloody mucus when swallowing the juice from chewing dulse. How do I know whether I would be able to eat it from a raw diet even if it is from juicing?*

A: The obvious solution is to avoid chewing dulse. Dulse contains too much salt to consume as a regular food item. Many people have cured or improved their colitis by consuming raw food and abstaining from irritating standard foods, like grains, meat, and dairy.

Do not compare juicing fruits and vegetables to the "juice" of dried dulse when eating it. Fruits and vegetables are water rich and not harmful to the esophagus or the digestive tract.

Durian and Digestion

Q: *I was wondering what your opinion is of the durian. I'm in love with it, but I think it is quite digestively challenging.*

A: I love durian, too, and, yes, it can be a little challenging to digest. The trick is to never mix it with anything else and have plenty of water before or after you eat it. I also think that the kinds of durians that we get in the Asian stores are not ideal. I traveled to South-East Asia and tried different kinds of durian. Not only do they taste much better, but they are also easier to digest than our imported durians.

Frozen Durian as a Staple

Q: *I am really dying for some advice. Getting good quality fruit is really hard sometimes, especially getting variety. I love frozen durians imported from Thailand. I have even been eating it as a staple, because I can get them pretty cheap (only 79 cents per pound). I like to eat a lot of durian, because it's sweet and not acidic. I've been trying to avoid too much acidic fruits, because my tooth enamel is damaged. Especially in the winter, most of the local fruits are acidic, such as kiwis, citrus, etc. The only problem is that I heard durians are irradiated! Have you heard this? Do you think eating frozen, irradiated durians as a staple (like, every day) would compromise my health?*

A: In my opinion, frozen durians cannot be a staple of any diet. I know for a fact that they are heavily sprayed with toxic chemicals. Perhaps those chemicals don't make their way into the fruit flesh because of the tough skin, but I'm not sure of it. I wouldn't be surprised if they'd be irradiated as well.

The other problem is that the fruit is frozen. I do not consider frozen fruits to be fresh foods. Sure, I do eat them occasionally, but they are not optimal, especially if they are eaten cold. Eating cold (frozen) fruit is the equivalent of putting an ice pack in the stomach. All digestion stops, and indigestion follows.

But, even if you eat your frozen durian fully thawed, it is still no longer a fresh food and in my opinion only fresh foods can be the staple of the diet.

Also, durians are high in fat compared to other fruits, and they are actually not available (in season) year round. This is a good indication that it's not meant to be eaten all year long either. Bananas can form a good staple for a raw diet during the winter. Organic bananas are inexpensive (if bought by the case), and they are not irradiated. In the winter, I eat bananas, apples, and pears, but I also eat other fruits as they are available. Persimmons become a staple until January. I also eat some citrus, but I wait until the end of the season (March) when oranges are really ripe and sweet. I eat yellow kiwis, which are not too acidic. Starting from April, we get good mangoes. If you want to rebuild your enamel, make sure you consume at least one pound of green vegetables per day, avoid all dried foods (including nuts and dried fruit), and a good dental hygiene routine.

Eggs

Q: *Many times I have read the same question being asked, namely about eggs consuming. This is why I am still reluctant to order your books. I am looking for a natural human diet. Let's ignore the controversial meat issue. But what wrong with eggs? Humans and apes always consume eggs. I am going 100% raw from mid-August (my birthday). I am desperately looking for an answer.*

A: It depends if you're looking at it from an anthropological perspective or a health perspective. Some people try to guess what the ideal diet is simply by looking at what humans have eaten, in the past, or what other apes eat. To me, that only tells part of the story.

The real question is:

• Are eggs truly healthy?

• Is there something in eggs that you cannot get from fruits and vegetables?

• Are there any concerns with eating eggs?

I can see a few things wrong with eggs. First of all, they are very high in protein, and a high-protein diet wears down the kidneys and contributes to cancer. High protein diets also are a major contributing factor in osteoporosis.

Eggs are also very rich in methionine, a sulphur-containing amino acid. That means they are very acidifying, because methionine is broken down into sulphuric acid by the body. That sulphuric acid delivers a big acid load to the body that must be neutralized by leaching precious calcium from your bones.

According the Relative Acid Load chart (also called Potential Renal Acid Load), eggs are some of the most acidifying food there is. Egg yolk is even more acidifying to the body than beef or salami. That goes for your raw eggs too.

There is also the potential of bacterial contamination with eggs. Many people have been seriously harmed by eating contaminated eggs, especially raw eggs.

Egg eaters live shorter lives. A recent study showed that men who eat more eggs live shorter lives: http://www.redorbit.com/news/health/1334002/eating_too_many_eggs_could_bring_early_death/

Since you can get all the nutrients you need from fruits and vegetables (except for the Vitamin B12 that is made in your guts. If you're concerned, take a supplement.), I see absolutely no reason to eat eggs, especially regularly, and many more reasons to NOT eat them.

Flax Seeds

 Please inform me if flaxseed is healthy for the human being. If so, please explain how to prepare it for the best assimilation.

 Flax seeds contain some goodies: essential fatty acids, minerals, etc.

Those nutrients can also be found in a variety of foods: other nuts and seeds, green vegetables, etc.

Flax seeds eaten whole are not digested. They are eliminated in the stools almost intact.

To be able to digest them, you need to either blend them or grind them first.

I'm not against flax seeds. Some can be beneficial, but they're not necessary for a healthy diet. I don't recommend flax oil at all.

Frozen Foods

 What's your stance on frozen foods?

When you address the issue of frozen foods, you perhaps miss the point that some of us thaw the food to room temperature before ingesting it. I find thawed frozen berries to be a most useful thing in wintertime for smoothies. And I have even heard it argued by certain highly-researched raw family members, that because these berries and such are flash-frozen soon after being picked, that they may even be more nutritious than fresh berries (or okra or whatever) that have been transported hundreds of miles, only to sit under fluorescent lights for a few days. Alas, we do our best.

A: I do not recommend frozen foods, except on special occasions. When fresh food is available, we should choose it instead. Frozen food is damaged by the cold, but the main problem is that they are consumed cold. You're right, the problems with frozen foods are not as great if those foods are consumed thawed. However, most people eat those berries frozen, in smoothies, for example. Freezing destroys approximately 15-30% of vitamins. But the main thing to remember is that frozen foods are no longer "fresh". They are always second choice. But, you're right; we do our best!

The Garlic Issue

Q: *I get your newsletter regularly, but I have tried to research further regarding the toxicity of garlic. The only article I can find is the same one that you mentioned. Frankly, I don't know if I believe it. There doesn't seem to be any comment or further research on this 10-year-old article. Have you done any personal study on this? Don't know if I'm ready to give up my garlic just yet.*

A: Toxicity is a big word. Garlic contains some compounds, which are extremely strong. However, most garlic in the world is consumed cooked, so these compounds are destroyed in the cooking process. In addition to that, people do not generally consume large amounts of raw garlic due to the related problems of breath and digestion.

I cannot point you to specific studies that have been done on the "toxicity" of garlic, because they do not exist. There is no point for researchers to spend time researching garlic, while there are bigger issues out to research!

My point of view on garlic is based on basic logic that any 5-year old can understand. Garlic is so strong that you would never want to eat it in its natural state alone. It is used as a flavoring agent to stimulate the taste buds. After its consumption, every pore of the body smells like garlic. The breath is terrible to those who don't eat garlic.

Garlic is a "food" that has been avoided by natural hygienists for more than 100 years and for good reasons. We do not need any "study" to prove this.

However, if you want the specific names of the compounds in garlic that are considered to be irritants, the scientific names are: diallyl disulfide, allylpropyl disulfide, and allicin.

In conclusion, the garlic issue isn't a big one. I do not want to make a big fuss about it. It seems to me more obvious that we shouldn't eat foods that have a really strong taste - foods that we could never enjoy in their natural taste if we didn't mix them with something else.

Personally, I absolutely hate garlic breath, and that's the main reason that I avoid it: to spare my loved ones of it!

On a more serious note, I also find that when I eat garlic, I can tell the fact that it's an irritant by the way my body reacts to it, but that's because I rarely eat any so that I'm not accustomed to it as some garlic eaters are!

Why Are Greens So Healthy?

 What makes the "green" in green vegetables and what is it in these green vegetables that are so good for you?

 Chlorophyll is what makes the green vegetables green, but it's not what makes them good for us.

Green vegetables contain more vitamins and minerals than all other foods. The calcium in green vegetables is better assimilated than the calcium in cow's milk as well.

Also, green vegetables contain an abundance of phyto-chemicals that help fight cancer and other diseases.

Goji Berries

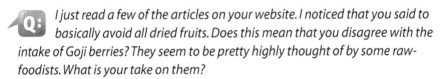 *I just read a few of the articles on your website. I noticed that you said to basically avoid all dried fruits. Does this mean that you disagree with the intake of Goji berries? They seem to be pretty highly thought of by some raw-foodists. What is your take on them?*

One thing with Goji berries is that a lot of claims are being made about its nutritional value, but I've never seen a complete nutritional analysis of those dried berries to back those claims up. So, as far as I'm concerned, there's a lot of hype surrounding this product, not to talk about the super-high markup on something that we basically only have heard rumors about.

There are many people claiming that they have the true Goji berry, and others are only selling the far inferior wolfberry that isn't grown or harvested in an organic way.

I've tried them, but I have not noticed any great benefits from them. Additionally, they're rather a hassle to soak before eating, because they're fairly dry.

Goji Berry Juice

Q: *What do you think about goji berry juice?*

A: I had the chance to try a bottle of Goji Berry Juice a while ago. For those who don't know, goji berries are a highly nutritive dried fruit that is sold as a "superfood". Now a multi-level marketing company is selling a product called "goji juice".

I must say that this juice is rather delicious. That's the good thing about it.

The rest: at $40 US a bottle, plus shipping, it's hard to find a better rip-off in the world of supplements. This "special" juice is nothing more than grape and apple juice mixed with reconstituted goji juice with a few artificial preservatives thrown in there.

On the bottle, we can read some ancient "legend" about the discovery of the goji berry in the Himalayans, and that's the only justification for charging this outrageous price for this ordinary juice.

As far as the health benefits are concerned, well, maybe there are some. But I'd rather spend my money on whole, organic fruits and vegetables instead.

The Goji Berry Hype

Q: *I recently attended a talk in Honolulu where a well-known, raw-food enthusiast touted the cancer-curing, life-changing, thought-enhancing, libido-strengthening Goji Berries. I bought some and tried them. They taste okay, but are they all that they're touted to be? Please let me know. Mahalo (thanks).*

A: They're okay, of course, for a dried fruit. I'm not big into dried fruits, so, if you could have other fresh berries, it would be even better. I don't attribute to them any particular property, but they're more nutritive and less dense in sugar than other dried fruits, so if you want to carry dried fruit on a trip, goji berries would be a better choice, because they don't get stuck to your teeth.

But libido strengthening? Sounds more like an old wives' tale to me. Didn't you say the guy who was raving about them was selling them?

Do salesmen really know what's best for your health?

Is Eating the Skin on Nuts Harmful?

Q: *Hi, I'm new to the raw food diet, and I have been doing some research about it, hoping to transition soon. I have a question about nuts and tannic acid. When I buy raw nuts in their shells and shell them myself, is ingesting the brown skin on the surface of nuts like almonds and Brazil nuts harmful due to its tannic acid content? I have heard this can compromise iron absorption. I have also read that removing the skins by soaking is possible, but, as this is inconvenient, I would like to know your thoughts on skipping this step, especially if I'm only having 60 grams of nuts a day.*

Thank you for all the work you have done to help others gain control of their health. Your book The Raw Secrets is by far the simplest, most straightforward book on the raw diet that I have come across, and it is definitely the one that makes the most sense!

A: It's not necessary to remove the peel from almonds and other nuts. The old books that recommended that you do this were written at a time when most of the almonds were imported from Spain and were of a much more bitter variety.

"Modern" almonds do not contain that much tannic acid, so it is safe to eat them. You might want to soak and peel them if you want to achieve a certain consistency and taste for a recipe. There's nothing wrong with that. But it's not necessary to avoid them for that reason.

Kale

Q: *I'm loving the green smoothies! My question is about using kale. I've read some stuff now that suggests avoiding cruciferous greens, because they aren't digestible and can cause an acidic condition. What are your thoughts?*

A: I've never heard about that. Green vegetables, on the contrary, are quite alkaline. The issue with kale is more digesting it, due to the rough fiber. So I find it's best to use it in small quantities only, blended in green smoothies, after carefully removing the stem, which is too hard to digest and very bitter.

I don't use it in salads because it's very hard to chew and must be wilted with salt and oil first which kind of defeats the purpose of eating it for its health benefits.

Kombucha Tea

 Could you please address the use of Kombucha Tea while on the raw foods diet? Is it good or bad?

 I'm really surprised that so many people make the mistake of eating a particular food or taking a particular product because of the alleged health benefits. Why not pursue a healthy lifestyle as a whole?

Kombucha Tea does contain some caffeine, although certainly not as much as regular tea or coffee, depending on what kind of leaves it's made from. But it is a good enough reason to avoid it.

This tea is also fermented, and it will generally contain a certain percentage of ethyl alcohol, formed through the fermentation process. That also is another reason to avoid it.

There are also possible adverse reactions when a culture can become contaminated through the fermentation process.

On the other hand, I don't really see any serious health benefits from drinking Kombucha tea, as most claims made about its health benefits are either dubious or simply not proven.

Some claim it helps their digestion. It's already fermented and unnatural to eat fermented foods, so it's no wonder the body expels this soon after ingesting. The same happens when you get food poisoning: the body rushes it out of your system. It doesn't mean it's helping your digestion.

I find eating fruits and greens to be the best way to improve digestion and absorption on the raw food diet.

So I really see no reason to drink it, especially not for health benefits.

Papaya Seeds

Q: *Many thanks for all the information. Is it okay to eat papaya seeds?*
They are sort of bitter, but I was wondering if the seeds have health benefits.
Please advise. Thank you.

Aren't you supposed to do things to get rid of parasites? I thought it was okay to
eat things that occur in nature (such as papaya seeds) to cleanse your body of
parasites. There is much to learn. Now I'm REALLY confused.

A: According to T.C. Fry, the first rule of eating is, "Thou shall not poison
thyself." There is absolutely no reason to eat papaya seeds. They are a bit
poisonous, and, in fact, in many countries they are used to force a miscarriage.
Papaya seeds also reduce the potency of male sperms in animal species.

The main problem and source of confusion that I see are when people are
trying to use certain foods as *medicine* instead of what it should be used for:
a source of nourishment.

If you make raw fruits and vegetables the main staples of your diet, you do not
need to fear parasites under most circumstances. If you do this and find out that
you have parasites, then maybe a natural or even allopathic remedy might be in
order. Ask yourself, though, why are you trying to medicate with food or drugs
before you know there is a problem?

Would you take some aspirin every day, before you had a headache?

Would you take antibiotics every day, before you had an infection?

If not, then why do so with the same with foods that are clearly NOT foods but
"remedies" (and often unproven ones).

Also, papaya seeds taste extremely bitter and spicy. If you enjoy eating them
that way and can make an entire meal out of them, then go for it.

I know for sure that I couldn't do that, and most other people couldn't either.

If you want nourishment, eat the edible portion of the fruit. The rest is not
meant for your consumption.

Sun Tea

Q: *I was wondering if Sun Tea (which is made by putting a tea bag in a jug of water, then letting it set in the sun for a few hours) would be an acceptable beverage for somebody who wants to adapt a raw food diet. At least in my part of the world, the temperature of the water would never exceed 115 degrees Fahrenheit, and the tea leaves are dried, so I don't see any cooked element in it. Of course, there is some caffeine in some teas, but you could also make it from an herbal "tea" with no caffeine. I'd be extremely interested in hearing your opinion on this in an upcoming blog post.*

A: I don't see anything majorly wrong with that. I personally avoid all forms of caffeine and would recommend that you do the same for optimal health. Your health is your own, so, if you choose to include some sun tea in your diet for your enjoyment, then so be it.

Young Coconuts

Q: *One question for you: what do you think of young coconuts? Are both the water and the flesh okay to eat? Thanks for your work. It is really appreciated.*

A: I think young coconuts, when bought in tropical countries, are fine foods. The water is refreshing and full of minerals, and the meat is easy to digest. However, young coconuts sold in Asian stores in North America have been sprayed with a toxic substance, and the tips are dipped in formaldehyde. According to my tests, this can actually reach the water. (Just put a young coconut from an Asian market in a solution of water and food dye, and you'll see the dye will reach the coconut water and change its color too.)

So I advise you to consume those Thai coconuts from the Asian markets only occasionally. If you live or travel to countries where fresh coconuts are available, then have them as often as you'd like!

How Did Primitive Man Open Young Coconuts?

Q: *Do young coconuts belong in the raw food diet? I cannot imagine how primitive man could open them without tools. What do you think? Thanks.*

A: Yes, young coconuts can be a nice addition to a raw diet. It's possible to open them with only rude tools, such as sharp rocks. Even monkeys do it. I've personally had the experience to try that when I was traveling in tropical countries!

The younger they are, the easier they are to open, if you can cut and peel off the green shell it's not too hard to open the coconut inside.

Nowadays most people use a machete or sharp knife to open them quickly in the tropics. You can also get coconut openers online which allow you to make a hole in them and insert a straw.

The 10 Deadliest Mistakes Made by Raw-Foodists

And How Avoiding Them Can Take Your Health to a New Level!

by Frederic Patenaude

The following report has been published on my website and features an overview of my raw food approach. It is featured in these last pages for easier reading. To learn more about the raw food diet, make sure to grab a copy of my Raw Health Starter Kit, available at
www.rawstarterkit.com

#1: Eating a High Fat Diet

Not understanding the relationship between fat, protein, and carbohydrates is a common reason for failure on a raw-food program.

One should understand that there are only two main sources of energy: **carbohydrates and fat.** In a raw food program, cooked complex carbs are restricted or eliminated. This includes: bread, pasta, potatoes, cooked grains, etc. Healthy carbohydrates are then limited to one main source: **fruit.**

The other significant source of energy comes from fatty foods, which would be: nuts and seeds, avocados, and oils. In a typical Standard American Diet, fatty foods comprise more than 40% of caloric intake, which is widely recognized as unhealthy. In some raw diets, where not enough fruit is consumed to provide the bulk of energy needs, the caloric intake coming from fat can be up to 80%!

Why is that? **It's simply because of the fact that vegetables are not a significant source of energy (calories).** Thus, if not enough fruit is consumed, one will invariably find himself over-consuming fatty foods in the form of nuts, seeds, avocados, and oils.

This overeating of fats may lead to several problems: fatigue, skin problems, lack of concentration, weight gain (or even excessive weight loss), failure to thrive, sensitivity to fruit sugar, diabetes, hypoglycemia, candida, feeling "spacey", and more.

The solution to this is to completely **redesign the menu.** The first step is to limit fat to about 10% to a maximum of 20% of daily calories, while at the same time eating more fresh fruit to meet our energy needs.

To do this, we need to understand several things:

- The relationship between fat, carbohydrates, and protein

- How many calories we need in a day

- How many fatty foods it takes to reach the 10-20% limit

- What fatty foods should be consumed

All of these and more are answered in my book The Raw Secrets, included in the **Raw Health Starter Kit.**

For now, let's just say that a healthy, raw-food program that provides about 2000 calories per day should contain, as a maximum:

- One small avocado, OR

- A small handful of nuts, OR

- 2-3 Tablespoons of nut butter

#2: Under-Eating or Not Consuming Enough Calories

Calories are a measure of energy, that is, how much energy is derived from the foods we consume. Only three components of food can provide calories (energy): **protein, carbohydrates**, or **fat**. The two main sources are **carbohydrates** and **fat**, as protein is mostly used for repairing and building tissues.

Raw vegetables are low-caloric foods. They contain very small quantities of fat or carbohydrates. Although they are excellent sources of vitamins and minerals, we cannot make them the basis of our diet, or the source of our calories (energy). It would be impossible to consume enough of them to meet our needs.

Raw Fats, which include avocados, nuts, and seeds, are good foods when consumed in small quantities. As we have seen, a high-fat diet is disastrous. Limiting the quantities of fats in our diet is essential for achieving success. Therefore, we cannot regard raw fats as our main source of energy. They should be used only as completing sources.

Raw Fruit is a healthy source of carbohydrates in the form of natural simple sugar. The obvious conclusion from this discussion is that it should form the basis of the diet, in terms of providing our calories. Raw fruit is easy to digest, contains an abundance of vitamins, and is not as concentrated as cooked carbohydrates or fatty foods. Therefore, it requires some calculations and some work to learn to eat enough fruit to meet our energy needs on a raw-food program.

Many people who try to follow a raw-food program are on a starvation diet. That is, they consume much less calories in a day than they spend. That program can be good for a while, to help detox, weight loss, etc., however, in the long run, it won't be sustainable.

#3: Eating Insufficient Quantities of Greens

Although fruit is a great source of energy and vitamins, it doesn't contain enough minerals to be a balanced food. Green vegetables must be consumed to provide those essential minerals, such as calcium, magnesium, sodium, etc.

Most raw-food programs do not contain sufficient quantities of green vegetables required for optimal health. Many raw-food programs that promote eating large quantities of nuts and seeds do not contain sufficient quantities of vegetables. The fact is, when we eat a salad with oil and fats, there is less room to eat enough green vegetables. But, when we eat a low-fat diet, composed of fresh fruits AND vegetables, there is more room and hunger to eat enough of those important foods.

It must be stressed also that greens should be consumed in a way that is easily assimilable by the body. Just eating a salad of greens might not be enough, unless it is carefully chewed. That is why I promote eating blended greens (either as a "green fruit smoothie" or as a "raw soup", as well as some vegetable juices, occasionally).

#4: Not Paying Attention to Food Combining Rules

In addition to containing ridiculously high quantities of fat, most raw-food programs will give you complicated recipes where foods are often dehydrated or mixed in every possible way, resulting in mixtures that lead to all sorts of digestive problems.

I call these recipes "combo-a-bombs" — that is, they are "combinations" that are "abominations"!

Although in a raw-food program, the issue of food combining is greatly simplified, the use of some simple food combining principles can help to ease your digestion tremendously.

After all, eating simple foods in their natural state should be the focus of a raw-food program, don't you think? Trying to imitate regular Standard American dishes with raw dishes is a recipe for confusion and can lead to sheer abuse.

Simple Food Combining Rules to Follow

Sugar and Fat

The main combination to avoid is sugar and fat. Sugar is any type of sugar, such as fruits, dates, refined sugar, or anything sweet. Fat includes oils, avocados, nuts, and any other type of fatty foods.

The reason is that fat takes a longer time to digest, while sugar tends to digest quickly.

When the two are mixed together in sufficient quantities, the sugar will ferment. Say hello to gas and bloating!

So the combinations to avoid include: dates and nuts, nuts and dried fruits, adding fat to fruit smoothies (including oils, nuts, etc.), and, obviously, eating fruit or sweets at the end of a meal.

However, let me also say that although this is the most important rule to follow, it is not completely rigid either. A little, occasional combo of fruit and fat are okay, but, generally, you'll find that avoiding this combination most of the time will solve a lot of your digestive problems.

Sugar and Starch

Another very bad combo is the combination of cooked starch and sugar, so this one obviously doesn't apply to a raw food meal. Starch includes bread, potatoes, pasta, etc.

This combination leads to a lot of gas and fermentation. Examples include: raisin bread, all pastries, all cakes, all cookies, and eating sweets after a meal.

Concentrated Foods

You can understand the philosophy and science of food combining by understanding one simple idea: it's best to eat only one type of concentrated food at a meal.

Concentrated foods include anything that's not a fresh fruit or vegetables, or anything that's high in fat. For example, bread, meat, potatoes, nuts, seeds, or avocados.

The reason is that concentrated foods take more time to digest, and, when they are mixed together, they tend to conflict with each other and cause digestive problems.

So the idea is that in one meal to have just one type of concentrated food, and accompany that with lots of vegetables. It's also best to eat fruits alone.

Unnecessary Rules

There are several "rules" of food combining that are really not necessary. Once you become more fluent in the "language" of food combining, you'll understand why. Let me give you a few:

Melons - There's no reason not to mix melons with other fruits. You can mix melons with any other fruit you want, without any problems. Just don't mix them with concentrated foods.

Fruits - Fruits may be combined with each other without problems. There's no need to divide them in categories of their own. The only exception is the banana, which should not be mixed with very acidic fruits, such as oranges. The reason is that bananas contain starch and that conflicts with the acidity in certain fruits.

Tomatoes - Although we eat tomatoes as a vegetable, it is a fruit in reality, so it may be combined with other fruits if desired.

Greens Don't Count – Greens, such as lettuce, celery, spinach, and other green leaves, don't even count in food combining. The reason is that they combine well with anything. They combine well with fruit as well as with any other food.

#5: Having a Fanatical Approach

It is too common in the raw-food movement to see people completely obsessed with their diet, over-stressing it, and forgetting about the other important aspects of life. Some want to feel "pure" at all cost, and they think that all cooked foods are evil. Yet, at the same time, they will not hesitate to consume large quantities of avocados, nuts, seeds, and "combo-abombos", thinking that just because it's raw, it's okay!

"Raw" is not the only criterion. It doesn't mean that because something is raw it's healthy. Most of the raw-food recipes that I've seen are actually not healthy at all! They contain large quantities of salt, spices, oils, and fat.

Instead of just focusing on the "raw" aspect and forgetting everything else, let's try instead to go back to the basics, which is to eat "whole foods" — fruits and vegetables in their natural state!

Personally, I prefer to eat steamed vegetables rather than all sorts of heavy, nut-based, raw-food recipes. But some raw-foodists still like to think that it's okay to eat a few jars of almond butter in a week, as long as it's raw almond butter. They don't realize that they are actually setting themselves up for all sorts of problems with that sort of narrowed-thinking.

Let's go back instead to the basic principles of a natural diet, before even thinking about raw or cooked. (I have outlined those basic principles in my book *The Raw Secrets: The Raw Vegan Diet in the Real World*)

Let's also not forget about the other aspects of healthful living. Diet isn't everything. Did you know that there are at least 21 requirements to healthful living, and any one missing will hold you back to achieving the level of health that you desire?

Here are just some of those requirements, besides good food and nutrition:

- Securing enough sleep
- Sunshine
- Pure air
- Pure water
- Regular physical activity
- Sense of belonging to a group

- Natural expression of sexuality
- Fulfillment in the professional life
- Adequate temperature
- Beauty in surroundings
- Self-expression of natural talents
- Sense of connectedness to family members and friends

#6: Eating Many Spices and Condiments

We're designed to eat foods in their natural state, just like every other living creature on the planet does. Therefore, eating a natural diet doesn't just mean eating "natural" foods or eating "raw" foods, but it means eating those foods "whole" and unrefined.

One of the things humans love to do is adding spices, salt, and condiments to their foods. Why do we do it? Simply because of the fact that we're out of touch with nature and our natural diet, and because we get USED to eating condiments and salt, as those substances are habit-forming and slightly addictive.

What are the problems related to the regular consumption of spices and condiments? First of all, they are all slightly irritating. They are all foods that we couldn't eat in their natural state (ever think of making a meal out of raw garlic?).

That substance may be the strong irritant oil found in hot peppers, or the pungent mustard oil found in garlic, or any of the other irritants found in all of the spices consumed.

All of those spices stress the body, disturb digestion, and prevent us from enjoying the natural taste of foods. The more we use them, the less we will enjoy foods in their natural state.

Unfortunately, most raw-food programs do not understand this and promote eating a lot of cayenne pepper, raw garlic, sea salt, soy sauce and other condiments. They simply copy the wrong eating habits of the SAD and transfer it to their raw-food program!

Yet, everybody who has done the experiment of abstaining from salt and condiments for an extended period of time will tell you that the enjoyment that they get from eating foods in their natural state actually increases! Soon, the strong taste (and smell!) of condiments becomes offensive, and it is no longer desirable.

Try it out for yourself.

That being said, you can still use minimal quantities of certain spices (especially the mild varieties) in a recipe for taste, but, overall, they should be minimized.

#7: Doing Insufficient Physical Activity

Physical activity is one of the requirements of healthful living. It is actually so intricately linked with optimal nutrition that failure to master one aspect will automatically lead to failure with the other.

While fitness alone is not a guarantee for health, it is not possible to be healthy without being fit. We must learn to develop our fitness potential by including a variety of exercises into our lifestyle, in a complete program that builds and trains our bodies.

Engaging in vigorous physical exercises (each to his/her ability) will also help create genuine hunger, which is one of the first requirements for optimal nutrition.

It will help sugar uptake (or metabolism), overall nutrition, and improve our sense of well-being, self-esteem, and more!

Let's also stress the fact that a raw-food program is actually a high-energy diet. It is compatible and really works only with a high-energy lifestyle.

Of course, each will train according to his/her own abilities and limitations. But by making your fitness an aspect as important to master as proper eating will insure that you don't overlook this most important aspect of healthful living.

#8: Forgetting About Dental Hygiene

A careful plan for taking care of your teeth, preventing decay, and other problems is absolutely essential while on a raw-food program or any other program. Yet, many raw-foodists forget that, thinking that "raw foods can't be bad for their teeth", and they end up with severe dental problems.

Why go down the same road? A complete dental health program doesn't take a lot of time, and it will save you lots of trouble.

The use of non-toxic dental products, as well as proper brushing, flossing, gum irrigation, tongue cleansing, and a good diet are essential.

#9: Consuming Raw Drugs & Unneeded Supplements

Having boundless energy should be the natural outcome of a healthy lifestyle. It doesn't come from eating certain foods, taking certain products, or using supplements. When it does, then it means that the product or food you are taking is a stimulant — a drug — not a real source of nourishment.

Raw drugs are now popular in raw-food programs. They include the now much hyped raw cacao, which is the "raw" version of chocolate; and, in addition to probably not being really raw (the cacao beans are fermented at a high temperature before being sold as "raw"), it is addictive, disturbs sleep patterns, and is just another way to take your dose of caffeine or the equivalent.

Other raw drugs include various supplements and superfoods that are sold for their "energy-boosting" properties, just like various caffeinated drinks are sold for the same purpose. Energy doesn't come from stimulation, but it can only come from sleep and as the outcome of healthful living.

Of course, the profit markup from selling those foods is more than nice, and their addictive nature hooks the customer up and invites repeated sales — not bad for the company selling it, but not good for your health.

If you are not experiencing the levels of energy that you desire on your raw-food program, it is time to revise it entirely, rather than resorting to some sort of raw stimulant.

#10: Eating Too Many Dried Fruit & Dates

Dried fruit is the junk food of the raw-foodist. As we've seen, people, eating a raw-food diet that is too high in fat and not eating enough of the caloric-rich foods, end up hungry and try to fill up on something. Dried fruit is often that "comfort food" that people revert to.

Dried fruit is fruit with the water removed. Thus, it is no longer a whole food. It is extremely sweet — too sweet — and is notoriously known to cause gas, fermentation, and dental problems. I've known for a long time that eating dried fruit causes extreme cravings for other junk foods. The reason is that because dried fruit is a concentrated sugar, it disturbs digestion entirely and causes one to become extremely imbalanced in their sugar-metabolism. Thus, they crave other foods, in that state of nutritional confusion.

Dried fruits are also refined, often frozen in advanced, and/or dried at a high temperature before they are shipped to the stores. Although dates are can be fresh, they are too concentrated to form an important part of the diet.

I recommend phasing out dried fruit and dried dates and instead eating them occasionally, only, as a treat or when circumstances call for it (like a trip to a foreign country, camping, etc.). I guarantee that you will feel much better.

To make sure that you don't crave dried fruit, eat enough fresh fruit instead. If you eat enough fresh fruit there is no way that you can crave dried fruit.

Conclusion: Get the Right Information

If you were to buy a car, would you just buy any model right away without even thinking about it, or would you research the subject thoroughly before making a decision? I'm sure you would spend a lot of time analyzing the different options before making the right decision.

Yet, when it comes to their health, many people are careless. They search the Internet, looking for quick fixes, and read free articles. They try to make sense of it all by asking complete strangers for health advice in a random bulletin board. They do not take the subject seriously.

This is how they hurt their health unnecessarily, like I did when I first started on the raw food diet without knowing what I was doing.

That's why I've created the **Raw Health Starter Kit.**

I've wanted, for a long time, to put together a kit of resources that would give anyone everything they would need to successfully switch to a raw food diet, include more raw food in their diet, or improve their current raw food program.

It took me over 8 years of research to put together all of the resources that are included in the Raw Health Starter Kit, and, in fact, I keep updating it all the time with new information.

When properly done, either at 100% or 70% level, the Raw Food Diet can bring you the following benefits and more:

- Gives you amazing energy. You wake up in the morning ready to go, and you rarely feel ups and downs in your energy during the day.

- Improved complexion. People will comment how clear your skin is.

- Reach your ideal weight effortlessly.

- No feeling of deprivation.

- Great sleep and no insomnia problem.

- Regular bowel movement and with no constipation or indigestion.

- Looking younger than most people of your age.

- Clear and bright eyes

- Makes you happy for no reason. You don't need coffee to stimulate you or alcohol to make you laugh.

  Better focus and concentration.

If you are not experiencing all of these benefits, then it's time to revise your current program.

If you purchase the Raw Health Starter Kit, you'll get everything you need to get started on raw foods (or improve your current program), including:

- My best-selling book, The Raw Secrets: The Raw Vegan Diet in the Real World"

- My course, How to End Confusion about Nutrition

- My recipe book, Instant Raw Sensations

- My DVD Series, "The Low-Fat, Raw Vegan Cuisine (three DVDs)

- My menu planner, Best Foods on the Planet

- Tons and tons of other bonuses and resources not available anywhere else. That totals over $400+ in REAL value.

Here's what one of my readers had to say about the Raw Health Starter Kit:

"After having a mixed experience eating all-raw foods and reading numerous websites and cookbooks about the subject, I decided to give the Raw Health Starter Kit a try.

I was skeptical after participating in some other raw food programs, including a local delivery service. Although I felt a million times better than when I was eating cooked food, I was still getting sleepy and sluggish at times.

The Raw Health Starter Kit is honestly the best money I've spent going raw, and I wish that I had found this website first. I think Fred's observations and advice are spot-on and the way to be a healthy, supercharged raw-foodist.

His recipes are fantastic and incredibly simple; even my non-raw fiancé has taken to making some of the salads and smoothies.

Perhaps the best thing about Fred is that he is non-dogmatic about raw food, and, at the same time, his system is firmly rooted in science and practical common sense. Anyone who wants to eat more raw food would definitely benefit from this kit, not just raw-foodists. Given how poor the nutritional information is out there, I recommend this to anyone who simply wants to eat better.

Danica Radovanov
From Los Angeles,
California, USA

Here's another letter I recently received:

Dear, Frederic,

Hi! I'm 53 years young and getting younger. I ordered the Raw Health Starter Kit about a month ago, and I am really enjoying all the great information and recipes contained therein.

4 months ago, I found out that my blood sugar was through the roof! My cholesterol, blood pressure, and triglycerides were all out of control. I had been taking pills for several years to "control" these things. I was tired of just covering it up, knowing good and well that I could do something about it.

Well, that pushed me right into getting healthy. The great thing is now that I am eating raw and exercising. It just, overall, gets easier, because I feel better than

I have in years. As part of my recovery, I started reading everything that I could online about true, healthy living that I found your site and all the other free information, so I decided to get more info. I ordered the Raw Health Starter Kit to give me more specific info and more motivation.

There are so many recipes, tips, and general good health info that I am still reading, acting on, and then reading more and again. I really like having both the e-books/files, hard cover books, and CDs.

Well, I have been monitoring my blood pressure and sugar levels, went to my doctor for cholesterol and triglyceride levels, as well as A1C (long term sugar level), she has taken me off all those harmful chemical meds, because every level is in the excellent zone.

I look better and feel better. I want to get out, and exercise my body. All the fruits and veggies taste so clean and wonderful. I went out to dinner with the family and ordered just a raw veggie salad no dressings, cheese, etc.

Had a little craving for what they were eating, but seeing all the oils, salt, grease, and fat just reminded me of how poorly most people in the world eat.

Also, I knew that if I didn't cave into false desires and went to bed that I would be glad in the morning. True enough, the next morning those cravings from the night before had no emotional hold on me, and I was glad that I woke up light and healthy.

Thank you for your inspiration and easy-to-digest information programs. They are helping me stay the course and motivating me to do great things in my life.

Don Webber
From Encino,
California, USA

Here's another story from a reader in Australia:

Dear, Frederic,

Since ordering the Raw Health Starter Kit, life has definitely changed for the better. I am 61 years old, thought that I was eating well, and was a bit dubious about such a different way of eating. However, I gritted my teeth and began to follow the eating pattern that you recommended.

In only a few weeks, I noticed that I no longer had hot flashes, my asthma had disappeared (I no longer take any medication which I was taking for 14 years), and the arthritis in my hands vanished. I have noticed too that the liver spots on my hands have faded and are now almost non- existent.

When I did the pinch test on my hands, previously, the skin stayed erect, but now it goes back down immediately. I feel as if there is a glow about my skin. Additionally, the dentist has commented that my teeth are in better condition. I highly recommend the Raw Health Starter Kit for a healthier, fitter, and longer life.

Ann
From Australia

You'll find many more testimonials on the Raw Health Starter Kit, great success stories, and **before and after stories** of people who have completely transformed their life with the raw food diet on my website.

In fact, recently, we even completely redesigned the Raw Health Starter Kit to offer an even more complete package.

I won't try to convince you anymore about it.

Go to www.rawstarterkit.com and learn more.

I hope that you've found this book useful. I certainly would have benefited if someone had written it when I first got started, as this information was not available back then.

I'm looking forward to adding your story to our long list of success stories from people who have successfully applied the teachings in the **Raw Health Starter Kit!**

Wishing you health and success,

Frederic